KATE VAZQUEZ

Estrogen

IS A

B*tch

Break the cycle of menstrual agony to embrace sexy confidence, enhanced libido, happy periods and optimal energy with balanced hormones!

Contents

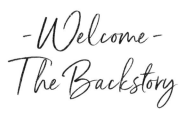

- Welcome -
The Backstory

I'm so excited you are reading this book! You're either at the beginning of your journey, or you already know about the basics of hormonal balance and want to dive deeper. Wherever you are, welcome!

Many women are suffering every month (or every two to three months if they have irregular cycles). Perhaps you're in this boat. One day I started thinking about Estrogen Dominance.

Two years after starting Radiant Health, I'd seen a lot of different hormonal imbalances. Finally, a pattern began to emerge, and I began to see what was happening.

Women came to me after being told their PMS symptoms were normal. Other providers told them their low libido was because they were tired, anxiety was from stress, and acne was just hormonal or genetic. Their blood work was normal, but they didn't feel normal and knew something was wrong.

These women were right!

Something was wrong!

Their bodies had imbalances in their gut, adrenals, and hormones, which caused them to suffer every month.

As a Physician Assistant, I learned from the conventional western medical model, which taught me that these symptoms are normal. They're treated with different prescription medications to manage the symptoms.

Most of the time, the treatment for hormonal imbalance is birth control (or hormonal contraceptives). But, unfortunately, birth control does not treat the root cause of why there are imbalances with the hormones.

Birth control suppresses your body's ability to produce sex hormones such as folliclle stimulating hormone (FSH), lutenizing hormone (LH), estrogen, and progesterone. Instead, it increases a protein called sex hormone-binding globulin, which binds up most of your testosterone. Later, I will discuss more about this and birth control's long-term effects that medical providers rarely discuss.

After taking birth control pills for over 15 years and stopping them to prepare my body for pregnancy, I started having symptoms of estrogen dominance such as breast tenderness and longer cycles between periods which I never had before.

I knew these symptoms were not normal. After hormonal testing, I discovered that my estrogens were too high in ratio to my progesterone, and I had low testosterone levels. I kept doing more research and learning about my body which helped me uncover that I have a genetic mutation of the COMT and MTHFR genes. This decreases my liver's ability to metabolize estrogen.

Why is this important?

It means I needed liver support with DIM, milk thistle, alpha-lipoic acid, and folate, as well as magnesium to help metabolize estrogens. As you continue to read, you'll understand why.

As I began to brainstorm how excess estrogen or estrogen imbalance affects the body, one phrase popped into my mind.

"Estrogen is a b*tch!"

Now mind you, I wouldn't say I like to use curse words and don't use this word lightly.

I surprised myself when I thought of this phrase! But then, I realized how appropriate it was to describe what women are experiencing and that I personally could relate to this as well.

After all, the term "b*tch" often describes an aggressive or dominant woman.

It also describes a woman who believes in herself to the extent that she does what she wants, even if others around her do not agree.

Either way, I do believe that estrogen has been misunderstood for years. Issues arise when there is too much estrogen in your body or when estrogen is out of balance.

When I thought of the title for this book, I realized I wanted to educate women about Estrogen Dominance. I want you to learn how to balance your hormones to no longer suffer every month.

Do any of these symptoms sound familiar?

* Mood swings
* Headaches
* Difficulty losing weight

* Severe menstrual cramps
* Irregular periods
* Trouble becoming pregnant

These symptoms all stem from estrogen imbalance.

My goal for you is to have more energy, mental clarity, and confidence, so you feel sexy in your body! In addition, I want you to achieve the health you deserve.

The overall message I want to portray is that estrogen is not bad at all. We need estrogen, which I'll dive into later, but estrogen does become an issue when it is not balanced and becomes a "b*tch."

So please don't find the title of this book offensive. Instead, use it to develop a deeper understanding and appreciation of the power estrogen has in your body and how it impacts the quality of your life.

Now let's get started!

Part 1

WOMEN HAVE ED TOO

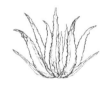

Chapter 1

WHEN ESTROGEN DOMINATES

Just like men have ED (also known as erectile dysfunction), women can have ED. But, in our case, it stands for Estrogen Dominance.

Estrogen Dominance means that the ratio of estrogen levels in your body is higher compared to progesterone levels.

There should be a balance between estrogen and progesterone depending on the specific phase of the cycle you are in, especially the luteal phase (the second half of your menstrual cycle after ovulation).

During the luteal phase, estrogen becomes the dominating hormone if you have a higher ratio of estrogen to progesterone. This is what contributes to many symptoms of Estrogen Dominance.

I will dive into the phases of the menstrual cycle at the end of this section. Too much or too little of specific hormones can cause hormonal imbalance and drive all the symptoms you're trying to eliminate! Therefore, I want you to have a greater understanding of the fluctuations of your hormones throughout the menstrual cycle.

When I started functional medicine, I didn't realize how prevalent estrogen dominance was in women (and men).

Western Medicine taught me that when women have severe PMS symptoms, we treat them with NSAIDs (think Advil, Aleve, or Midol) for pain and inflammation. Then, we turn to anti-anxiety or antidepressants for mood swings and hormonal contraceptives to control the hormone imbalances.

Nothing was ever mentioned about why this happened, only how to treat the symptoms with a prescription.

Conventional western medicine teaches as if it's normal for women to experience these symptoms. Testing is only done to rule out hormonal imbalances such as:
* Polycystic Ovarian Syndrome (PCOS)
* Endometriosis
* Dysfunctional Uterine Bleeding
* Fibrocystic Breasts
* Uterine Fibroids

But did you know that all these conditions stem from Estrogen Dominance?

Other Common Conditions of Estrogen Dominance:
* PMS/PMDD
* Short Luteal Phase
* Breast, Endometrial, & Uterine Cancer

ESTROGEN DOMINANCE IN MEN

Did you know that men can also have estrogen dominance like women?

Men produce estrogen in their bodies as women do, just in smaller amounts. In fact, erectile dysfunction can be caused by estrogen dominance.

If too much estrogen builds up in their bodies, not only will they have erectile dysfunction, but men can also have infertility, insulin resistance, enlarged breasts, enlarged prostate, and weight gain in the abdomen.

Estrogen dominance occurs when a protein called Sex Hormone Binding Globulin increases. This protein binds up sex hormones, primarily testosterone.

Estrogen is also made from testosterone by an enzyme called aromatase. Factors such as stress, alcohol, weight gain, and inflammation can increase the activity of aromatase. In the end, it causes the body to produce more estrogen, and the vicious cycle continues.

Men don't get their estrogen levels checked as a standard practice. Estrogen testing only occurs when symptoms of estrogen dominance appear. One such symptom is gynecomastia or enlarged male breasts. According to the Mayo Clinic, imbalanced testosterone to estrogen ratio triggers gynecomastia.

Let's flip this around!

The ratio of estrogen to testosterone is greater because testosterone levels are too low, which creates estrogen dominance. Other symptoms of excess estrogen in men include:
* Obesity
* Metabolic Syndrome
* Diabetes
* Enlarged prostate
* Increased risk of prostate cancer

Once again, conventional western medicine fails to address the underlying reason for this occurrence. Possible reasons for male estrogen dominance include genetics, lifestyle choices, and environmental factors.

Conventional western medicine tells men to avoid soy products because they contain weak estrogens. However, there's no mention of how dairy and red meat also have added hormones that can increase estrogen in their body. I'll discuss more about this later.

Would you like to know how conventional western medicine treats conditions like gynecomastia, erectile dysfunction, or an enlarged prostate?

First, there's the infamous Viagra for erectile dysfunction. But men are also prescribed anti-androgens. For example, Finasteride blocks the enzyme that converts testosterone to DHT (dihydrotestosterone). Other treatments include:
* Testosterone blockers like Spironolactone
* Aromatase inhibitors like Anastrazole, Femara, and Aromasin block the conversion of testosterone to estrogen
* Estrogen blockers such as Tamoxifen (commonly prescribed to female breast cancer patients)

* Anabolic steroids, which are a synthetic form of testosterone
* Androgens such as testosterone itself
* Steroid alternatives such as HCG
* Anti-anxiety and anti-depressant medications

Young men with low testosterone levels are given testosterone replacement which is not the right approach. In these cases, there could be something wrong with the reproductive system or an issue with the brain sending signals to the reproductive organs. A common cause of low testosterone in young men is STRESS. Checking the adrenal glands is helpful in these cases.

I believe that stress is the biggest and longest-running pandemic our country is facing. Most people aren't even aware of the severity of stress in their lives.

Why treat the symptoms with testosterone without addressing the underlying cause?

Some men even undergo surgery to remove excess fat, breast tissue, and glands. But, unfortunately, it can reoccur.

Why?

Because the underlying cause of estrogen dominance wasn't addressed. It's like putting a bandaid on a symptom and hoping it goes away without finding out why the symptom exists in the first place.

If you know any men experiencing these issues, please get them checked out by a functional medicine practitioner.

WHY DOES ESTROGEN DOMINANCE OCCUR?

Although there are several causes of estrogen dominance, the three most important are poor gut health, toxins, and birth control.

Poor Gut Health

Most of us have issues with the gut, whether we have gastrointestinal symptoms or not. Common causes of gut imbalance include:

* Processed or inflammatory foods you eat
* Medications you take or have taken
* Nutritional deficiencies
* Infections
* Environmental toxins
* Constant daily stress

The health of your gut plays a role in estrogen metabolism. Your body is responsible for using estrogen, then getting rid of it. Poor gut health can prevent this from happening. I will review estrogen metabolism in the next chapter. I will also dive more into gut health in Part II.

Toxins

I believe another cause of estrogen dominance is the overload of toxins. Toxins are everywhere! They're in the environment, toxic food, toxic chemicals, and toxic medications. We have toxic relationships and even toxic mindsets, which we develop over time because we live in more of a toxic world than ever before.

These "toxins" negatively affect our genes and our hormone production. In turn, this causes your body to produce either more estrogen, less progesterone, or both.

A study by the Environmental Working Group in 2005 looked at the chemicals of 10 babies' umbilical cord blood after delivery. They discovered 287 chemicals in the cord blood of these newborn babies! The chemicals came from pesticides, household products, and environmental wastes.

They also discovered that women use on average 12 personal care products per day. For example, lotion, toothpaste, body wash, shampoo, and deodorant contain about 168 ingredients.

The study found that men use fewer products, about 6 per day. But, on average, they're exposed to about 85 ingredients. Remember, this is from personal care products alone. It doesn't include the chemicals from household cleaning products, cookware, plastics, or pesticides from yard maintenance. It also doesn't involve chemicals in food, such as hormones and antibiotics or chemicals used in food processing. Other toxin exposure not included in this count results from exposure from chemicals at work, off-gassing from our furniture, paint, projects in the home, and so much more.

If this doesn't open your eyes to our toxic environment, I don't know what will!

When learning about all the toxins in the environment and in my home, I remember feeling overwhelmed. Finally, it got to the point that I wanted to move to an island and make everything homemade or live in a bubble! But then, I realized neither was realistic.

If you're starting to feel the same, don't worry! At the end of the day, the best you can do is decrease your toxic burden and support your body's ability to detox from all these chemicals.

Birth Control
Another common cause of estrogen dominance is birth control.

More women are on birth control than ever for several reasons:
* It's easily accessible.
* It's western medicine's answer to hormonal imbalance.
* It's a convenient way to avoid pregnancy as women take on more roles.

Birth control contains synthetic forms of estrogen and progesterone, but they suppress your body's ability to make your own hormones.

Studies find that birth control affects your gut microbiome. It also alters your liver's ability to make bile which reduces your body's ability to get rid of excess estrogen and metabolize it efficiently. I'll dive more into the effects of birth control on your body and how it contributes to estrogen dominance at the end of this section in Chapter 4.

I'll address the all of the main causes of Estrogen Dominance in this book which include:
   * Poor Gut Health
   * Poor Estrogen Metabolism
   * Medications (birth control/hormonal contraceptives)
   * Implantable devices (breast implants)
   * Histamine Intolerance
   * Excess Body Fat
   * Lack of Exercise
   * Stress

REDUCING YOUR TOXIC LOAD

When it comes to estrogen dominance and your toxic load, the good news is that you have a choice!

Start by shifting out of living a toxic life by decreasing your toxic load. Learn about the products you use and the food you consume. A great resource is the Environmental Working Group. You can start swapping out products you use and consume for healthier options.

Reflect on which relationships nurture you, and which relationships are toxic. Then, make a decision to set boundaries. Removing unhealthy relationships from your life can be difficult in the beginning. However, it's worth it in the long run because it helps your body to heal.

The most important shift is in your mindset and how you take care of your body moving forward. I won't dive much into mindset here because that is a book on its own. However, I will touch upon it as we focus on self-care of your body in Part III.

Talk to your medical provider about birth control and the long-term side effects that could occur. You have a right to know and decide what you feel is best for your body before choosing to take it.

Finally, supporting your body's detoxification will also help you to remove toxins. Sometimes toxin exposure is outside of your control. Supporting your body in healthy detoxification will prevent toxins from building up. I'll go over how you can support detoxification at the end of this book.

ESTROGEN: DEMYSTIFIED

All sex hormones, including estrogen, are made from cholesterol. So, like cortisol, they're classified as steroid hormones.

Estrogen is created in your body by your ovaries. However, it's also made in smaller amounts in your adrenal glands, liver, heart, fatty tissue, muscles, bones, and brain.

I don't want to give estrogen a bad rep because estrogen provides so many benefits when it's balanced. Here are a few of the roles estrogen plays in your body:
* Imparts womanly curves
* Plumps your skin
* Improves your memory
* Keeps blood vessels flexible
* Increases HDL (good cholesterol)
* Strengthens your immune system and bones

As I mentioned before, estrogen doesn't cause issues unless it's too high or too low. For example, when women go through menopause, estrogens decline. As a result, the skin loses elasticity, so it may sag and wrinkle, weight gain can occur, and memory isn't as sharp. There's also an increased risk of developing chronic disorders such as heart disease, Alzheimer's, diabetes, and osteoporosis.

Does this mean we should be scared of aging? No! I believe aging women are beautiful. Furthermore, proper hormone replacement therapy can help slow or reverse these effects.

So if aging by itself isn't the problem, then what is?

It's aging plus our toxic environments and lifestyles!

This book is dedicated to educating you on symptoms of high estrogen. In addition, it gives you helpful, easy-to-understand suggestions to restore balance to your hormones and your life!

TYPES OF ESTROGEN

Next, let's review the different types of estrogen your body makes from puberty through perimenopause. Perimenopause is the time just before menopause.

Did you know your body makes four different types of estrogen? When I first learned about hormones in high school, I thought it was just one... estrogen. Then when I dove into medicine, I was amazed to learn about all the different types of estrogen that our body creates.

Estrone
The first estrogen is called estrone, aka E1.

Estrone is actually a weak estrogen that helps with the development and function of female sexual organs. Therefore, it is usually not a problem in small amounts. However, it causes many problems when there is more estrone than other types of estrogen, which I will reveal next.

Estrone has the reputation of the "bad" estrogen because women with breast or endometrial cancer tend to have high levels. Also, women who are obese produce more estrogen from the adipose or fatty tissue.

Too much estrone combined with lower testosterone levels in men can contribute to prostate cancer. So I like to think of estrone as "the Rebel". When there are more of these rebel estrogens, there are more imbalances and disorders in your body.

Estradiol

The second type of estrogen is estradiol or E2. It should be produced in greater amounts than the other two estrogens.

You can think of estradiol as the "good" estrogen because it helps mature your reproductive organs. It also works in developing and releasing the egg during ovulation. Your body produces estradiol from testosterone and a little from estrone. However, estradiol can convert back into estrone.

Many women tend to make more estrone than estradiol, meaning they make more of the "bad" estrogen than the "good" estrogen. We will discuss more about why this happens when I review estrogen metabolism. It is vital to support the production of more "good" estrogen than "bad."

For now, think of estradiol as the Yogi...peace, love and abundance! When estradiol is in abundance, everything is balanced and functioning correctly.

Estriol

Estriol, aka E3, is the third type of estrogen that gets produced in tiny amounts. It is not detectable through regular blood work and is a weak estrogen like estrone.

Estriol is a "good" estrogen like estradiol because it has anti-inflammatory effects. In addition, studies show that estriol is also protective against cancer due to its antioxidant effects.

Free radicals get produced from metabolic reactions in the body when combined with oxygen. These molecules are unstable and react easily with other molecules. Therefore, antioxidants like estriol help to neutralize free radicals.

The placenta produces estriol, and levels increase during pregnancy. For this reason, some women with autoimmune disorders go into remission during pregnancy. Unfortunately, after pregnancy, estriol levels go back to their baseline, and autoimmune symptoms return.

Even though it's not easily detected in blood work, urine tests are made that accurately measure estriol levels. The DUTCH test or Physician's Labs can test all three of these estrogens.

Think of estriol as Wonder Woman who comes in to save the day and gets rid of those free radicals.

Estetrol

The last estrogen that gets produced is estetrol, or E4.

Estetrol is a weak estrogen and is only produced during pregnancy. The fetus's liver creates estetrol, and then it passes into the mother's blood-stream. Few studies exist to explain why fetuses make this hormone. However, a 1975 study suggests that estetrol is a good indicator of well-being in mothers with preeclampsia or chronic high blood pressure during pregnancy.

Estetrol has both estrogenic and anti-estrogen effects. Studies examined its usefulness as a hormonal contraceptive and hormone replacement in menopause. Unfortunately, these studies haven't been successful in either case.

ESTROGEN DOMINANCE PATTERNS

Over the first 2.5 years of practicing Functional Medicine, I treated many women with estrogen dominance. The more women I treated, the more I began to see different patterns emerge. Of course, most women presented with similar symptoms, but I began to see these patterns unfold when I ordered testing.

It became essential to understand these patterns because they determined the treatment. Not all types of estrogen dominance are treated the same. Let's dive into the three patterns of estrogen dominance that I discovered.

Estrogen Dominance #1:

For the first pattern, ED-1, women have *normal* progesterone levels but *high* estrogen levels.

Estrogens normally increase leading up to ovulation, then start declining. Then progesterone peaks around days 19–22 of a regular 28–day cycle.

If someone has this pattern, the progesterone peaks at its normal range. However, estrogens are also higher than usual instead of declining.

The leading cause of ED-1 is poor gut health, toxins, heavy metals, xenoestrogens, and genetics.

Estrogen Dominance #2:

The second pattern, ED-2, revealed *low* progesterone levels and *normal* estrogen levels.

With ED-2, progesterone doesn't reach its peak around days 19–22. This creates an estrogen dominance effect. Optimal ranges of progesterone should be between 15–25 during its peak. If it is 10 or less, this is usually a sign of low progesterone.

I usually found this pattern in women with nutritional deficiencies such as B6 and Vitamin C. These women were also stressed to the max. But, overall, they did not have too many gut issues. Their liver was keeping up with the metabolism of their estrogens.

This is the least common pattern of estrogen dominance that I typically see in women.

Estrogen Dominance #3:

The last pattern I discovered was ED-3. It features characteristic *low* progesterone and *high* estrogen levels.

With ED-3, progesterone doesn't peak around days 19–22 like ED-2, and the estrogens are higher than normal instead of declining. I usually see this in women who have a wide range of issues: nutritional deficiencies, high stress, poor estrogen metabolism, toxins, xenoestrogens, and genetics.

This is the most common pattern I see in my practice.

SYMPTOMS OF ESTROGEN DOMINANCE

How do you know if you have estrogen dominance?

The symptoms women experience aren't being diagnosed as estrogen dominance. Instead, these symptoms are often given diagnoses for other hormonal imbalances with similar symptoms such as:
* Polycystic Ovarian Syndrome (PCOS)
* Premenstrual Dysphoric Disorder (PMDD)
* Endometriosis
* Dysfunctional Uterine Bleeding
* Uterine Fibroids
* Fibrocystic Breast Disease
* And more!

These are the common symptoms of Estrogen Dominance:
* Irregular periods
* Heavy bleeding (with or without clots)
* Severe menstrual cramps
* Mood swings (anxiety, depression, irritability, anger)
* Breast tenderness and/or Fibrocystic breasts
* Uterine fibroids
* Bloating
* Acne
* Weight Gain

* Low Libido
* Painful Intercourse
* Hair Loss
* Insomnia
* Brain Fog
* Hot Flashes
* Fatigue
* Infertility

Out of all these symptoms, 5 symptoms are the tell-tale signs of estrogen dominance.

These symptoms are **irregular periods, heavy bleeding, PMS, breast tenderness, and weight gain**.

If you have two or more of these symptoms, there is a high chance you have estrogen dominance.

ED SYMPTOMS EXPLAINED

Irregular Periods
Irregular periods are a sign that there is an imbalance with your hormones.

The most common cause of irregular periods is Polycystic Ovarian Syndrome (PCOS) and endometriosis. Unfortunately, most women are unaware of the connection.

In PCOS, irregular periods are due to an excess amount of androgens. These include testosterone and DHEA (the precursor to testosterone). Excess androgens prevent the release of the egg from the ovary, so ovulation does not occur.

In addition to high androgen levels in PCOS, you may have excessive estrogen in ratio to progesterone. Of course, this hormonal imbalance often isn't addressed unless a woman is prescribed birth control which suppresses her hormones.

If progesterone is already low, birth control definitely doesn't fix the problem!

Your body relies on the fluctuations of your hormones. It sends signals to your brain and your reproductive organs to prepare an egg for release. They also signal the endometrial lining to shed when pregnancy doesn't occur, which triggers your period. Hormonal imbalance hinders these signals, stopping ovulation and menstruation.

How does this work?

High estrogen levels combined with low progesterone prevents egg release at ovulation. This postpones your period because your progesterone levels don't rise and decline as they should in the luteal phase. The result is a very irregular menstrual cycle.

Heavy Periods

The second sign of estrogen dominance is heavy periods, whether regular or irregular.

On average, you should only lose about 2–3 teaspoons or 30–50 ml total of blood in 3–7 days. Heavy bleeding occurs when you lose a total amount of 5 teaspoons or 80ml of blood. These periods may last longer than 7 days.

Estrogen thickens the lining of your uterus, called the endometrium. This prepares your uterus for pregnancy. However, excess estrogen causes the lining to thicken more than usual.

During ovulation, one ovary releases an egg. If it is not fertilized, progesterone and estrogen levels drop back down to baseline levels. At this point, your uterus begins to shed the endometrium and your period begins.

Women with a thicker endometrium have heavier, more painful periods because of the excess estrogen. Not only is there heavy bleeding, but blood clots the size of quarters can develop. This happens with PCOS, endometriosis, adenomyosis, and dysfunctional uterine bleeding.

Premenstrual Syndrome

Premenstrual Syndrome (PMS) is common with hormonal imbalances related to estrogen dominance.

Symptoms begin a few days to a week before your period starts. They include:
- Severe menstrual cramps
- Irregular period cycles
- Breast tenderness
- Headaches
- Mood swings

Premenstrual Dysphoric Disorder (PMDD) is another diagnosis given to women. Unlike PMS, PMDD has more intense mood swings. It can also include:
- Anxiety
- Panic attacks
- Depression
- Anger
- Low energy
- Difficulty concentrating
- Food cravings
- Binge eating
- Insomnia

Unfortunately, women are not told why these symptoms occur. Instead, women are often advised that these symptoms occur because of "normal hormonal fluctuations" when hormones decline the week before their period. The typical treatment includes NSAIDs (such as Motrin), birth control, antidepressants, and anti-anxiety medications.

The truth behind these diagnoses is actually low levels of progesterone compared to high levels of estrogen. This imbalance causes these intense symptoms that can devastate a woman's life.

Breast Tenderness

The fourth common sign of estrogen dominance is breast tenderness.

Progesterone and estrogen are responsible for the development of the breasts. Yet, when progesterone levels are low or estrogen levels are too high, women experience symptoms. Breast tissue swells, connective tissue increases, and breasts become tender. Cysts may also occur.

These changes explain why some women develop fibrocystic breast disease. Unfortunately, it may also increase the risk of breast cancer in some women. Later, when I explain estrogen metabolism, we'll talk more about what contributes to breast tissue growth.

Weight Gain

Weight gain is the fifth sign of estrogen dominance.

Hormonal imbalance affects the way your body distributes weight. For example, abdominal weight gain usually occurs from metabolic disorders such as insulin resistance, obesity, and diabetes. But, abdominal weight gain may also occur due to high cortisol levels from chronic stress and adrenal dysfunction.

Women tend to naturally carry some weight in their butt, hips, and thighs because estrogen naturally gives us our curves. Yet, women with estrogen dominance gain excess weight in their butt, hips, and thighs, making it a classic sign.

Some women with estrogen dominance don't experience weight gain at all. Others may have more of an issue with water retention. Women tend to retain more water with estrogen dominance which contributes to weight gain. However, this type of water retention is more generalized and happens all over the body.

Progesterone acts as a natural diuretic. When progesterone levels are low compared to estrogen, your body retains more water.

Bonus Symptom: Acne

I want to add this last symptom as a bonus because most people don't realize that acne often has roots in hormonal imbalance.

Conventional medical treatment of acne is as follows:
* Antibiotics
* Birth control (to reduce excess androgens and estrogens)
* Androgen receptor blockers (male hormone blockers like Spironolactone)
* Vitamin A derivatives (retinoids)
* Acids like salicylic acid or benzoyl peroxide

Ready for the truth behind acne? Studies actually show that certain foods cause breakouts. High glycemic foods, meaning foods that cause your blood sugar to rise rapidly, are a culprit. Inflammatory foods such as dairy and gluten also cause issues.

If you have acne, it's essential to start with your gut. First, remove inflammatory foods and focus on improving your digestion. This will bring healing to your gut lining and allow healthy gut bacteria to repopulate.

Toxic skincare products featuring unhealthy ingredients can also trigger breakouts.

The next step is to swap out toxic skincare products for natural alternatives that do not irritate or inflame the skin or clog the pores. Once you address the gut issues and swap out your products, it's time to examine your hormones if you still have acne.

The most common hormonal cause of acne in the medical world is high androgens, such as testosterone and DHEA. DHEA is actually the precursor to testosterone.

High androgens are often seen in women who have PCOS. This increases oil production and leads to acne. It is possible for women to have high estrogen levels, with or without high testosterone, and suffer from acne.

Healthy detoxification through the liver is vital for toxin elimination. When this doesn't happen, toxins and estrogens build up and cause skin inflammation, resulting in acne.

ESTROGEN DOMINANCE QUIZ

Take this quiz if you have gotten to this point and still don't know if you have estrogen dominance.

Put a number 1 by each symptom you have and add it up for a total score.

- ☐ Trouble losing weight
- ☐ Weight gain in the butt/hips/thighs
- ☐ Breast tenderness/Fibrocystic Breasts
- ☐ Irregular periods
- ☐ Severe menstrual cramps
- ☐ Mood swings/irritable
- ☐ Anxiety/depression
- ☐ Low libido/decreased interest in sex
- ☐ Brain fog (can't remember/think clearly)
- ☐ Acne
- ☐ Bloating
- ☐ Constipation/Digestive issues
- ☐ Headaches
- ☐ Retaining fluid/feeling puffy
- ☐ Difficulty falling asleep/staying asleep
- ☐ Hot flashes
- ☐ Constant Fatigue
- ☐ Elevated blood sugar/Diabetes
- ☐ Trouble getting pregnant/had miscarriage(s)

Scoring:

* If you scored 5 or below, you are less likely to have hormonal imbalance from estrogen dominance.
* If you scored 6–10, you are somewhat likely to have estrogen dominance.
* If you scored 11+, then you are most likely to have estrogen dominance.

However, the only way to be sure if you have estrogen dominance or not is to follow up with a functional medicine practitioner. You'll need specialized testing to determine hormone levels during certain parts of your cycle.

Chapter 2

BEHIND THE SCENES
OF ESTROGEN METABOLISM

The main reason estrogen builds up in your body is because your detoxification pathways become blocked or slowed. These pathways help to break down estrogen, eliminating the excess from your body.

When this happens, excess estrogen gets recirculated back into your bloodstream. As all this extra estrogen begins floating around, your body creates more receptors so the estrogen has somewhere to go.

Your body's ability to metabolize estrogen depends on a few factors:
* Nutritional deficiency
* Alcohol consumption
* Medications
* Toxins
* Inflammation
* Obesity
* Smoking

THE 3 PHASES OF ESTROGEN METABOLISM

Estrogen metabolism has three phases.

Phase I and Phase II, primarily occur in your liver. In Phase I, the estrogens are still in their active form, but they start to change into a water-soluble inactive form once they move through Phase II.

Following Phase I and Phase II, your body eliminates the broken-down components (also called metabolites) either through your urine or by binding them to bile. Phase III occurs in your intestines, where excess estrogens bound to bile leave your body with other solid waste via a bowel movement.

Phase I

In Phase I, estrogen goes through a process called hydroxylation. This means that estrone (aka "bad" estrogen or The Rebel) gets broken down into three different metabolites that have their own personalities.

The first metabolite is 2-hydroxyestrone (2-OHE1) and is The Protector. When Phase I is working efficiently, you produce more of 2-OHE1. This actually helps protect your DNA and decreases the growth of breast tissue cancer cells, reducing your risk of breast cancer.

It's essential to have higher levels of The Protector (2-OHE1). You can help your body produce more of this helpful form of estrogen by:
* Eating more cruciferous vegetables (broccoli, cauliflower, bok choy, cabbage, and kale).
* Taking high-quality fish or algae oil.
* Adding soy, rosemary extract, and flaxseed into your diet.

On the other hand, some lifestyle factors decrease the production of The Protector. For example, sugar and alcohol consumption reduces your body's production, so it's best to limit consumption of both.

The second metabolite is 16 alpha-hydroxyestrone (16a-OHE1). It's nicknamed "The Fertilizer" because it is like Miracle Grow for your cells.

The Fertilizer increases the growth of certain tissues in your body, such as breast tissue. It has an affinity for binding to estrogen receptors in the breast. When there is too much of this form, it can rapidly increase the growth of cancer cells in the breast, possibly leading to breast cancer.

16a-OHE1 is usually elevated when issues such as the following exist:
* Gut imbalance
* Hypothyroidism

* Obesity
* Toxic exposure to pesticides
* Too many omega 6's in your diet
* Increase in inflammatory cytokines

Healing the gut, regulating the thyroid, lowering inflammation, supporting detoxification, and losing weight will help decrease this form of estrogen.

The third metabolite produced from estrone is 4-hydroxyestrone (4-OHE1). When estrone transforms more into this type than the others, 4-OHE1 becomes The Destroyer and can damage DNA.

Breast, endometrial, and uterine cancers are all linked to this form of estrogen. It forms something called depurinating adjuncts, which change and damage your DNA.

The key to lowering 4-OHE1 are two compounds found in citrus and red skinned fruits: flavonoids and resveratrol. On the other hand, smoking and inflammation increase it.

You can also protect your DNA from damage by eating broccoli sprouts. This is because they contain sulforaphane, a powerful detoxifying antioxidant. In addition, eating foods like avocado and asparagus support your Glutathione S-transferase (GST) enzymes. GST enzymes also support Phase II of estrogen metabolism and protect your body from oxidative stress.

When you have low levels of 2-OHE1, and high levels of 16a-OHE1 and 4-OHE1, you've got the perfect storm and an increased risk of breast cancer.

This is why it is vital that every woman have her estrogen metabolites checked. I believe this testing can prevent a variety of estrogen-linked disorders such as:
* PCOS
* Endometriosis
* Adenomyosis
* PMS/PMDD
* Uterine Fibroids

- Fibrocystic Breasts
- Dysfunctional Uterine Bleeding
- Cancer (breast, endometrial, and uterine)

Phase II

Once the 2-OHE1 metabolite moves through Phase I, it goes through two pathways called methylation and glucuronidation. This is Phase II of estrogen metabolism, which occurs in the liver, creating an inactive, water-soluble form of estrogen.

What is fascinating is that these pathways are occurring in the mitochondria of our cells!

Methylation is the pathway that protects and repairs DNA. It is dependent on B vitamins such as Folate, Vitamin B12, and Vitamin B6 to convert 2-OHE1 into 2-methyoxyestrone (2-oMeE1).

Your body has an enzyme called Methylenetetrahydrofolate reductase (MTHFR). Suppose there is a mutation of the MTHFR gene that regulates this enzyme. In that case, it reduces the conversion of folic acid to folate, which can impact Phase II metabolism.

I have a mutation of one of the MTHFR genes (A1298C), because there are multiple (A1298C and C677T). For this reason, I need extra B vitamin support with Folate to boost Phase II metabolism.

Glucuronidation is the pathway that follows methylation. It is also responsible for producing water-soluble forms of estrogen and foreign chemicals, called xenobiotics, to be eliminated through our waste.

Many nutrients and cofactors help support and increase 2-oMeE1, such as Magnesium B6, B12, folate, betaine, and SAM-e.

Another enzyme called Catechol-O-Methyltransferase (COMT) helps convert 2-OHE1 into 2-oMeE1. However, it needs magnesium to support this reaction. Some women, like myself, have genetic mutations that slow down this enzyme. Therefore, we need a lot of magnesium to help it work effectively to increase the 2-oMeE1 metabolite.

S-Adenosyl-L-methionine (SAM-e) is also an essential cofactor in the methylation pathway. Your body creates SAM-e, and it helps support the production of 2-oMeE1.

Betaine is another important cofactor in methylation and is found in food such as beets, spinach, soybeans, and shrimp. Too much estradiol (E2) and rhodiola rosea can inhibit the production of 2-oMeE1.

Phase III

Phase III is the last phase of estrogen detoxification, and it occurs in your intestines.

Once estrogen goes through Phase II, the inactive forms are bound to bile or excreted through the urine. Your liver creates bile; it's stored in the gallbladder and released in the small intestine to help digest fats. It also plays a vital role in estrogen metabolism.

If women have disorders in the gut or with the gallbladder, estrogen is not eliminated. Instead, it gets reabsorbed back into circulation.

There is a specific enzyme in your gut that helps regulate estrogen metabolism called beta-glucuronidase. When you have a robust, healthy microbiome, this enzyme is low. This is because it allows the inactive forms of estrogen to get eliminated through our poop.

A disruption in your microbiome from an overgrowth of harmful bacteria, yeast, or parasites causes beta-glucuronidase to increase. This converts estrogen back into its active form.

Studies show that the food you eat can affect beta-glucuronidase levels. Foods that are high in animal and unhealthy fats, and low in fiber, increase levels of beta-glucuronidase. Conversely, foods that are higher in fiber help to lower beta-glucuronidase.

You now understand the metabolism of estrogen, the importance of each metabolite, and how each phase works. Each of these metabolites and the efficiency of the phases can be checked through specialty testing. Unfortunately, most conventional doctors do not order these tests, and they are not covered by insurance.

Knowing the status of your metabolites helps you:
   * To balance and optimize your hormones long term
   * Know which phase needs support
   * Reduce estrogen-related disorders and cancer

This means you'll no longer have to suffer from your symptoms, and you can overcome or prevent any estrogen-dominant disorder.

Most of these tests have to be (and should be) ordered by a licensed medical practitioner. You can work with them to help you find the best protocol for your body since there are different ways to treat estrogen dominance. I'll review these at the end of this book.

I recommend following up with a functional medicine practitioner or a naturopath. Request blood, urine, and a stool test to assess these pathways and metabolites.

At the time this book is published, the urine test is the best test to assess the Phase I and Phase II metabolites. The most common test used by functional medicine practitioners is called the DUTCH test, which stands for Dried Urine Test for Comprehensive Hormones.

There are other companies who can also assess these metabolites, such as Physician's Labs and Genova Diagnostics. The benefits of Physician's Labs is that they can bill your insurance first to try to get coverage.

The best test to assess Phase III metabolism of estrogen is a specialty microbiome test that checks beta-glucuronidase levels such as the Genova GI Effects or Doctor's Data GI Map.

Chapter 3

YOUR MENSTRUAL CYCLE EXPLAINED

PERIOD VS CYCLE

Before I dive into the menstrual cycle, I want to clearly distinguish these two terms. I notice that they tend to be used interchangeably but mean different things.

A period is the length of time that you are actually bleeding. The average woman will bleed anywhere from 3 to 7 days. If you are bleeding less than three days or more than seven days, this could signify hormonal imbalance.

A cycle is the total number of days from the start of one period to the next.

The average cycle length is about 28 days, +/- 1–2 days, but know that most women do not have a 28 day cycle. Women have a regular cycle when the amount of time is consistent between periods.

For example, the average cycle length is about 26 to 30 days between periods every month. So it is normal to be off a day or two between cycles, just not off by 7 or more days.

When women have an irregular cycle, it is a varying number of days between periods. For example, one cycle can last 37 days, the next cycle lasts 46 days, and the next lasts 32 days. Cycles like this are not normal. It means there is an imbalance in the hormones, such as too much estrogen and/or testosterone, and/or low progesterone.

MENSTRUAL CYCLE PHASES

Did you know that there are 4 phases of your menstrual cycle?

These four phases are the menstrual, follicular, ovulation, and luteal phases. They occur in one cycle, and on average, the total cycle lasts 28 days. However, the entire length of a normal cycle can be anywhere from 24–32 days. I personally believe that any cycle shorter or longer than that is due to imbalances in the hormones.

Let's dive into each phase of your cycle.

Menstrual Phase

The menstrual phase begins your menstrual cycle, which is the first day of your period (Day 1).

On average, women can bleed anywhere from 3 to 7 days. So, remember, if your periods are shorter than three or last longer than seven days, this could signify hormonal imbalance.

Some women may also have spotting a couple days before their period. This is normal and happens because of the decline of our hormones. However, spotting does not start the period. Your period starts when you have a full flow and need to use a period product such as a tampon, pad, or cup to absorb the blood.

Your period also starts the beginning of the follicular phase, typically lasting about 10–16 days on average.

During this time, all of your hormones, such as follicle stimulating hormone (FSH), luteinizing hormone (LH), estrogen, progesterone, and testosterone, are at a low baseline level. This is why you may feel like your energy levels are at their lowest.

Follicular Phase

The follicular phase is a two week timeframe beginning with your period and ending the day of ovulation.

On average, this occurs on days 1–14 of a 28 day cycle. However, it can be a little longer or shorter depending on your unique body. Once you finish your period, you'll have a few days where you are dry before your cervix starts to produce cervical fluid or mucus.

FSH starts to rise to help mature an egg in your ovary in preparation for release at ovulation. During the follicular phase, the endometrium (the inner lining of the uterus) also starts to thicken due to increasing estrogen levels.

Testosterone increases along with estrogen as well until both reach their peak right before ovulation. You may start to feel a rise in your mood and energy levels due to the rising of these hormones.

From days 8–16, your cervix starts secreting cervical mucus. The mucus prepares your vaginal canal by making it easy for sperm to swim past your cervix into your uterus. The end goal is for fertilization of the egg to occur.

On days 8–10 of your cycle, the cervix starts to produce mucus which is yellow, white, or cloudy and has a sticky or wet consistency.

Then, on days 11–13, this mucus becomes a white and creamy consistency just before ovulation. Your estrogen and testosterone levels spike as well. These higher estrogen levels cause LH (luteinizing hormone) to rise and peak 1–2 days before ovulation. This is what helps to release an egg from your ovary.

Have you noticed some days you feel confident, sexy, on top of the world, and get a boost in your libido?

This happens because of the spike in estrogen and testosterone right before ovulation. Your body is getting you ready for pregnancy, whether you want it or not, as this is your natural biology and body's rhythms.

Ovulation

Ovulation typically occurs on day 14 of a 28 day cycle. Depending on the length of your cycle, it could actually happen anywhere from day 12–17. At this time, your cervical mucus becomes clear and stretchy, like egg white consistency. You are the most fertile when this happens. These are the best days to conceive if you're trying to get pregnant.

You technically only have a 24-hour window to get pregnant each month. However, sperm can live in your vaginal canal for up to five days. It's important to know that you can still get pregnant up to five days leading up to ovulation if you are not using protection during vaginal sex during this time. Vaginal sex is the only way to get pregnant.

If you don't want to get pregnant, you have a couple of options during these six fertile days: don't have sex, use protection, or enjoy other forms of sex instead of vaginal sex.

Once an egg is released, estrogen, testosterone, LH, and FSH levels start declining. One to two days after ovulation, your mucus starts to change again, making it difficult for sperm to pass through your cervix. The fluid may turn back to that thick white creamy consistency, then to the yellow, white sticky texture, and dry again just before the cycle starts all over again.

Luteal Phase

The luteal phase occurs right after ovulation which is day 15 of a 28 day cycle. Depending on your cycle, it can start anywhere from days 12–17 if you don't have a standard 28 day cycle.

During your luteal phase, progesterone starts to increase because it is the pregnancy hormone. If an egg is fertilized, it moves through the fallopian tube and implants in your uterus. Progesterone is the hormone that maintains and sustains pregnancy.

Progesterone reaches its peak around days 19–22 of a 28 day cycle. If you have a regular cycle, you can also calculate it by subtracting 7 days from the total length of your cycle. For example, if your whole cycle usually is 30 days, your peak day is day 23.

This is when I like to check women's hormones. We can really see the amount of progesterone in ratio to estrogen, which is essential to assess in women with hormonal imbalance.

If pregnancy occurs, progesterone levels continue to rise. If pregnancy does not happen, then the egg does not implant into the uterus. As a result, your progesterone levels drop, and you'll start to feel a decline in your energy levels. Once progesterone reaches baseline with the other hormones, your cycle begins all over again.

MOON CYCLE SYNCING

Did you know that most women's bodies synchronize with the moon cycle? Moon cycles are an average of 29 days. So it makes sense why most women may sync with the moon.

Many years ago, when it was time for the new moon, women would get together under a tent to menstruate. This was called the red tent. They used this as a time for rest and self care so they could get back to providing for their families.

We should definitely take a page from their book in terms of self care during our period. Powering through the menstrual phase sets us up for burn-out!

These ancient women also knew that they were most fertile during the full moon, making it the best time for them to procreate. I thought this was fascinating and made sense because they didn't have apps to track their period and cycle back then!

Our modern society is filled with technology that disrupts our circadian and natural rhythms. In addition, we have more stress and increased exposure to toxins. As a result, women do not connect with each other or their bodies like they did before.

For this reason, some women do not sync to the moon cycle. This is especially true in those with irregular periods and those who use hormonal contraceptives.

If you have a 28 to 30 day cycle, you may notice you are cycling with the moon. Most women tend to menstruate around the new moon and ovulate around the full moon. This is known as the white moon cycle.

Other women are the opposite. They menstruate around the full moon and ovulate around the new moon. This is known as the red moon cycle.

You may find that neither applies to you. For example, perhaps you start your cycle between the new and full moon (the waxing or waning phase). Don't worry! As long as you have a regular cycle every month, this kind of cycle is entirely normal for you and not a cause for concern.

If you have an irregular cycle or a cycle that is shorter than 26 days or longer than 32 days, you can learn how to sync up with the moon cycle. This happens by doing seed cycling, which I'm excited to share with you in Part IV.

If you want to dive more into your menstrual phases, know when you ovulate, and when you can get pregnant or not, I highly recommend doing my online course called **The Estrogen Reset**. Please visit the website at www.yourradianthealth.com.

Chapter 4

THE TRUTH BEHIND BIRTH CONTROL

When you're not taking birth control, remember that estrogen peaks before ovulation. This helps to help mature an egg in your ovary in preparation for release.

As estrogen levels decline and luteinizing hormone (LH) begins to surge, the egg is released at ovulation. However, if too much estrogen exists in the body, it acts as natural birth control.

When you get a prescription for birth control, it contains synthetic estrogen. This hormone prevents your ovary from releasing an egg. It also keeps progesterone levels from increasing to avoid pregnancy.

There are synthetic forms of progesterone (called progestin) in birth control but in low amounts. You see, estrogen without progesterone thickens the endometrial lining and can lead to endometrial cancer, so you need both.

Synthetic estrogen and progestin also change the lining of your uterus to prevent the implantation of a fertilized egg. In addition, they transform your cervical mucus to prevent sperm from entering the cervix (the opening to your uterus).

There are many types of birth control, hormonal and non-hormonal. Hormonal birth control comes in the form of pills, patches, IUDs, rings, or injections. The non-hormonal form is the copper IUD.

Most women who take the pill usually experience bleeding during the last week of the pack. Did you know this isn't actually a period? This is actually a withdrawal bleed since those tablets do not contain any hormones. With the other forms, some women may not bleed at all because of the constant release of hormones.

LONG TERM EFFECTS OF BIRTH CONTROL

Unfortunately, women usually are not educated about the long-term effects birth control has on the body.

For example, you may or may not be aware that it can increase the risk of clotting. This can cause strokes and heart attacks, especially if you smoke or have a genetic clotting disorder such as Factor V Leiden.

Every birth control prescription comes with an excerpt that lists the possible side effects. However, what is not included in this reading material, is that it disrupts your microbiome, affects detoxification through the liver, and increases a protein called Sex Hormone Binding Globulin (SHBG).

SHBG binds up sex hormones such as testosterone, dihyrdrotestosterone (DHT), and estradiol but prefers DHT and testosterone over estradiol. This is why you may experience hair loss and low libido while taking birth control or hormonal contraceptives. In addition, your testosterone levels are low since they are bound to the SHBG protein preventing testosterone from being active in the body.

Birth control may help women with PCOS for this reason. It lowers your androgens due to SHBG increasing to bind up these hormones. However, the longer you take birth control, the higher your levels of SHBG. Therefore, you may continue to have high levels for years, or for life, after you stop using it.

I have personal experience with this. I took birth control pills for over 15 years to treat acne. I had low libido and was losing a lot of hair everyday. After I finally stopped taking the pills, my testosterone levels were so low that I worked to naturally increase them. Thankfully, my libido is back, and I'm not losing all my hair anymore!

In addition to increasing SHBG and lowering testosterone, birth control increases C-Reactive Protein (CRP), a marker of inflammation. It also increases insulin and triglycerides. In metabolic disorders such as insulin resistance, obesity, and diabetes, these markers are all increased.

Studies also show an increase in liver enzymes such as AST, ALT, and GGT, and even bilirubin levels are elevated when women take birth control.

Because of birth control's effects on the liver and gallbladder, it has also been linked to gallbladder disease such as:
* Gallstones
* Cholecystitis (inflammation of the gallbladder)
* Cholestasis (slow bile flow)
* Bile duct obstruction

Studies show that birth control decreases your liver's ability to make bilirubin which is important for bile production. In addition, as I have already discussed, bile helps bind inactive estrogen, which occurs during Phase II estrogen metabolism. This enables it to be eliminated through our poop in Phase III.

Also, progestin is found to slow down gallbladder motility. So if your gallbladder is not as active and becomes sluggish, bile accumulates in the gallbladder to form sludge. Then with the increased amount of cholesterol in the bile sludge, this makes for a perfect environment to make gallstones.

In fact, studies have shown that birth control increases the risk of gall-bladder disease. So women who have a prior history or develop any form of gallbladder disease while on birth control should not continue to take it.

As for your gut and microbiome, studies show that birth control leads to a "leaky gut" by increasing intestinal permeability.

Here's what this means:

Usually, the lining of your intestines is tightly closed. It only allows small particles such as water, electrolytes, and nutrients to go through the intestinal cells. However, many things cause damage to your gut lining, such as medications (NSAIDs and birth control), inflammatory foods, stress, and disruption of gut bacteria. This causes the tight junctions to loosen up, resulting in intestinal permeability. Basically, it allows holes to open, which enables toxins and microorganisms to pass through.

About 80% of your immune system is in your gut. When this happens, your immune system ramps up. This paves the way to developing auto-immune disorders, such as Crohn's or Ulcerative Colitis. Both are linked to increased intestinal permeability resulting from birth control.

If you are thinking about coming off birth control, I highly recommend also checking out Dr. Jolene Brighten's book "*Beyond the Pill*." In this book, she describes a condition she terms Post Birth Control Syndrome (PBCS).

Dr. Brighten discovered that about four to six months after stopping birth control, women developed symptoms such as:
* Acne
* Hair loss
* Severe PMS
* Headaches
* Mood swings
* Bloating

It was definitely a great resource for me when I stopped taking birth control after being on them for over fifteen years.

The information in her book works with what I am providing you in this book regarding hormonal imbalance and estrogen dominance.

Part II

DIVING DEEP INTO
ESTROGEN DOMINANCE

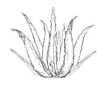

Chapter 5

ESTROGEN BALANCE AND GUT HEALTH—
A MATCH MADE IN HEAVEN

There are trillions of microorganisms in your gut that make up your microbiome, from bacteria, viruses, parasites, protozoa, and yeast.

These trillions of microorganisms present in the gut are more than all cells in your body. This is pretty fascinating when you think about it! You're literally outnumbered!

These microorganisms have many essential jobs in terms of overall health. In fact, one of the critical jobs for specific microbes in your gut is estrogen metabolism, which is also known as the estrobolome. This term comes from the combination of estrogen + microbiome.

When you have a disruption of the microbiome, such as an overgrowth of bacteria, yeast, or parasites, we call it dysbiosis.

When dysbiosis occurs in your gut, your microbiome increases an enzyme called Beta-glucuronidase. This enzyme is important in estrogen metabolism. It usually is present in low amounts to help estrogen metabolize out through our poop.

More estrogen is converted from its inactive form to an active, unbound state when this enzyme becomes elevated from dysbiosis. Then it is reabsorbed and recirculated in your body instead of being eliminated. This contributes to higher levels of estrogen, which results in estrogen dominance.

It is vital to assess gut health, because poor gut health impacts estrogen metabolism in Phase III.

I am commonly asked, "Can my primary care provider order a stool test for me?"

The answer is no. The stool test that they typically order, which is covered by insurance, is very basic and only helpful if you have an acute infection.

For example, if you recently took antibiotics or traveled to Mexico and developed diarrhea, this test can determine if you have an acute infection. Maybe you have an overgrowth of harmful bacteria such as C. Diff from taking antibiotics or picked up E. Coli or a parasite from Mexico.

This test does not look at the chronic overgrowth of bacteria, yeast, or parasites that may not cause acute symptoms but still impacts your gut health. It also assesses the amount of beta-glucuronidase you produce in your gut to determine Phase III estrogen metabolism.

I recommend following up with a functional medicine practitioner for specialty microbiome testing. Testing such as the Genova GI Effects or Doctor's Data GI MAP will determine if you have any dysbiosis from an overgrowth of specific microorganisms, inflammation and measure beta-glucuronidase levels to see if any of these markers are impacting estrogen metabolism.

BLOATING

Why do women experience bloating with estrogen dominance?

Bloating occurs for a few different reasons. The first is from water retention, as I mentioned previously. This occurs when progesterone is lower compared to estrogen.

Another cause of bloating is gut issues that slow down motility, causing constipation. Food does not get digested well and becomes fermented. This results in gas production, leading to bloating.

Remember, excess estrogen is supposed to get eliminated from your body through your poop.

When there are issues in the gut leading to slow motility or constipation, beta-glucuronidase increases so estrogen does not get eliminated. Instead, it is reabsorbed back into circulation, leading to higher estrogen levels in your body.

Lastly, histamines are a big issue that many people have and are unaware of that causes bloating in your gut. I'll talk more about Histamine Intolerance in Chapter 9.

SIBO

One of the common gut issues that causes bloating, slows down motility resulting in constipation, and affects estrogen metabolism is small intestinal bacterial overgrowth (aka SIBO).

Symptoms of SIBO include:
* Gas (I mean foul, rotten egg-smelling gas, which is NOT normal)
* Bloating
* Constipation or diarrhea
* Abdominal pain

I personally had experience with this and believe a majority of the population has this, as I have seen and treated about 80% of my clients for SIBO. First, however, we must understand the causes of SIBO or the overgrowth of bacteria into the small intestines.

Here are the causes of SIBO:
* Medications (antibiotics, antacids, birth control)
* Stress
* Low Stomach Acid
* Hypothyroidism
* Gastroparesis (Delayed gastric emptying)

* Diabetes
* Intestinal/abdominal adhesions

Each of these causes of SIBO disrupts your microbiome. In addition, they allow the overgrowth of bacteria into your small intestines, especially if low stomach acid is present.

When food enters your stomach from the esophagus, it's mixed with hydrochloric acid (HCL), which is acidic. HCL activates Pepsin, an enzyme that helps break down protein. This mixture of HCL and partially digested food becomes chyme or a ball of mush. Chyme leaves your stomach and heads into your small intestines.

Because this ball of mush is acidic, it creates an acidic environment in your small intestines, preventing intestinal bacteria from growing there. However, if you have low stomach acid levels, this environment is not acidic enough to control growth. Bacteria begin to take over, eventually leading to an overgrowth of bacteria in your small intestines.

Some bacteria that take over release gases such as hydrogen and methane. Specific breath tests assess if either of these gases exists after drinking a sugary solution called lactulose. However, these tests are not 100% conclusive or exclusive for SIBO.

Believe it or not, many people have heartburn or gastroesophageal reflux (GERD) due to having low stomach acid levels. Unfortunately, many people think these conditions originate from having high acid levels, but that isn't always true.

Of course, the conventional treatment includes an H2 histamine blocker or proton pump inhibitor (PPI) to suppress the release of stomach acid. But doesn't this sound counterintuitive if your stomach acid levels are already low?

There is a simple home test to determine if you may have low stomach acid levels, called the stomach acid test. When you drink baking soda mixed in water, it reacts with HCL in your stomach producing carbon dioxide. This should result in burping within a few minutes. If burping does not occur after 5 minutes, it is a sign of low stomach acid.

STOMACH ACID TEST

✳In the morning, before eating or drinking, mix ¼ teaspoon baking soda in 4–6 ounces of water.

✳Drink the solution and start the timer to see how long it takes to burp.

✳If you burp within 2–3 minutes, this means you have normal levels of stomach acid.

✳If you don't burp up to 5 minutes later, this could be a sign of low stomach acid.

GALLBLADDER DISEASE

Excess estrogen is a cause of gallbladder disease. Signs and symptoms include inflammation, infection, blockage, formation of sludge or stones in your gallbladder.

Earlier, I discussed how hormonal birth control contributes to this. When taking hormonal birth control, you are taking in excess estrogen through a pill, injection, IUD, ring, or patch. Studies show that women are twice as likely as men to have gallstones.

In the Physician Assistant program (and even medical school), we are taught that people who have the four F's: female, fat, fertile, and forty were more likely to have gallbladder issues.

Unfortunately, we were not told about the root cause of why this happens. I have now discovered that estrogen plays a huge role.

So how does estrogen cause gallbladder issues?

Studies show that estrogen increases biliary cholesterol secretion, which leads to more cholesterol in your bile. When high estrogen levels occur during the luteal phase, during pregnancy, or from hormonal contraceptives, there is more cholesterol in your bile to form gallstones.

Gallstones are made up of calcium salts, bilirubin, and cholesterol. Excess estrogen also increases bile acids leading to cholestasis, or a decrease in the bile flow from your liver. It is common in women who have estrogen dominant conditions, who take hormonal contraceptives or are pregnant. If you have had gallstones or gallbladder issues, it's time to get your estrogen checked.

ORAL AND VAGINAL YEAST INFECTIONS

Candida is a yeast that can exist in your body's microbiome, but only in small amounts.

The problem arises when it takes over, especially in your skin, gut, mouth, and vagina. Studies show that when Candida is exposed to estrogen, estrogen increases its growth and survival. This is why you may have vaginal yeast infections right before your period or during pregnancy. These are the times when estrogen levels are higher.

Estrogen helps your vaginal cells to produce glycogen. This is converted to lactic acid by Lactobacillus bacteria. The Lactobacillus species helps create an acidic environment to allow good healthy bacteria to grow. It also prevents harmful bacteria and yeast from taking over.

However, if the pH and environment of your vaginal canal become disrupted, Candida can grow. Factors that increase the risk of Candida overgrowth include:
- Antibiotic usage
- Overuse of hygiene products

* Douching
* High consumption of carbs and sugar
* Spermicides and other chemicals

Other studies show the link between vaginal Candida infections and the overgrowth of intestinal Candida. After all, your microbiome isn't just in your gut. It's in your vaginal canal as well.

Suppose the microbiome in your vaginal canal is impacted by excess estrogen (with or without hormonal contraceptives). In that case, we know there must be an overgrowth of Candida in your gut.

If you have or are currently taking birth control, have you ever had vaginal yeast or oral thrush infections?

If so, this is because birth control is linked to the development of vaginal and oral yeast infections due to excess estrogen.

Chapter 6

INSULIN: A VITAL HORMONE
NOT TO BE IGNORED

We've seen a rise in metabolic disorders such as obesity and diabetes due to:
* The Standard American Diet (which is high in animal protein, refined carbs, sugar, and unhealthy fats)
* Stress
* Sedentary lifestyles
* Genetics
* Decreased quality sleep

We can control most of these factors, except for genetics. However, even when it comes to your genes, you can still turn them on or off with your lifestyle and environmental choices.

As for sugar consumption, women shouldn't consume more than 24 grams per day which is 6 teaspoons (1 tsp = 4 grams). However, Americans eat an average of 22 teaspoons or more of sugar per day, about 88 grams, which is way too much!

Unfortunately, so many foods have added and hidden sugar. Even pack-aged foods that seem healthy include added sugar, so it tastes better. This entices people to eat more of it. When you eat sugar, it targets the dopamine receptors in your brain, your pleasure and reward center. Because sugar exists in so many foods, it adds up quickly throughout the day. I'll show you an example in Chapter 15.

Even though there are no studies that directly link estrogen dominance to insulin resistance, I believe there is an indirect link.

How does insulin resistance occur?

After you consume a meal, feel stressed, or wake up, your brain increases glucose in your body. Your pancreas then releases insulin to help lower those glucose levels.

If glucose levels remain elevated long-term, insulin resistance develops. This happens when your body becomes less sensitive to insulin. After time, high levels of insulin circulating in your bloodstream causes your body to ignore it.

We have also discovered that when people gain weight, their fat cells actually produce and release more estrogen. So I believe that this is another cause of estrogen dominance because of the extra estrogen created by fat tissue.

OPTIMIZING GLUCOSE

So how can we optimize our glucose levels?

Most people think they should go low carb or keto because carbs and sugar spike insulin, which is true.

However, foods that do not contain sugar tend to have added alternative sweeteners (acesulfame potassium, aspartame, saccharin, and sucralose) or sugar alcohols (erythritol, mannitol, sorbitol, xylitol, lactitol, isomalt, and maltitol) that can also spike your glucose.

I have had clients on a keto diet or who drank diet sodas have an increased glucose response, which shows why it's not for everyone. However, when we restrict carbohydrates, ketones do get formed as a source of fuel. This is the outcome people are after when going on a keto diet.

Some people don't realize that our bodies also use fat and protein, which turn into glucose as well.

A fat molecule is made up of one glycerol molecule and three fatty acids. When broken down, glycerol can be made into glucose via a process called beta-oxidation.

As for protein, there are a total of 20 amino acids. All except for two (leucine and lysine) can be turned into glucose via a pathway called gluconeogenesis.

Diets aren't one size fits all. We're all different. The best way to find out the best foods for your body that won't spike your glucose is through continuous glucose monitoring. This tool isn't only for diabetics. It has made its way into the biohacking world.

What is biohacking exactly?

It's making changes in your environment and lifestyle to optimize your health and longevity.

CONTINUOUS GLUCOSE MONITORING

In conventional western medicine, only diabetics check their blood glucose levels by doing a finger stick or using a continuous glucose monitor (CGM).

However, if most chronic diseases, such as heart disease, obesity, and Alzheimer's, are due to insulin resistance, why don't we all check our glucose response to food?

I believe we all should check our blood glucose, as this is one way to prevent these chronic disorders.

Another reason we should check is because we're all different, and our bodies react differently to the same types of food. For example, two people can eat a banana with almond butter. One person will have an elevated glucose response above normal. The other will have a normal glucose response within range, even though it is the same food and bananas are a higher glycemic index food.

Pairing a banana with healthy fat, such as almond butter, helps reduce the glucose response in some people, but not everyone.

INSTRUCTIONS FOR CGM

✳Check your fasting glucose as soon as you wake up in the morning. This should be after 8–12 hours of fasting through the night to get your baseline.

✳Next, check it an hour after eating each meal and snack, and document what you ate and your glucose level to see what foods are causing your glucose to spike.

✳Keep a log of what you are eating and to record your morning fasting glucose and glucose levels after eating.

Levels
After 8–12 hours of fasting in the morning, the optimal glucose range is 70–85mg/dl.

One hour after eating, glucose should jump no more than 30mg/dl.

For example, if your baseline is 80, it should not jump up over 110 an hour after eating.

>> Note: If you check it within 15–30 minutes, it is natural to see glucose levels higher because insulin hasn't taken effect yet. An hour after eating is enough time for your pancreas to release insulin and for it to work.

If glucose is greater than 30mg/dl an hour after eating, this could mean you had too many carbs and/or sugar. It could also mean that your cells are not responding to insulin to take it out of your blood to use it as fuel or store it in your liver, muscles, or fat.

If your glucose jumps up more than 30mg/dl, look at what you were eating to determine what could affect your glucose. Then, see if you can pair it with healthy fat, protein, and/or fiber or switch up the ingredients to get a lower response.

If it is >60mg/dl, this is too much spike and probably should be avoided.

If you continue to have readings >60mg/dl, I recommend following up with a licensed medical provider to rule out a metabolic disorder causing insulin resistance.

Recommended Monitors

These are the monitors available at the time this book is published.

FreeStyle Libre—requires a prescription from a licensed medical provider (MD, DO, PA, NP, or ND).

Dexcom—requires a prescription from a licensed medical provider.

Levels—does not require a prescription as they have their own medical providers. Find it at www.levelshealth.com.

NutriSense—does not require a prescription as they have their own medical providers. Find it at https://www.nutrisense.io.

HIGH CORTISOL AND GLUCOSE

Another indirect mechanism that can contribute to estrogen dominance is high cortisol levels in your body.

When you are stressed, your body goes from a relaxed, rest, and digest state to a fight-or-flight (or freeze) state. Rest and digest are controlled by your parasympathetic nervous system. Fight or flight is controlled by your sympathetic nervous system.

When cortisol levels are high, more glucose is released to fuel your muscles so you can fight or run. However, your body doesn't know the difference between stress from getting into an argument or facing a predator in a life-threatening situation.

I always tell my clients, our ancestors primarily lived in a parasympathetic state and only shifted to sympathetic in immediate danger.

Our modern world has constant demands for our attention. With our on-the-go schedules, we operate from a mostly sympathetic state. Our bodies were not meant to constantly produce cortisol all day long. Imagine the long-term effects on our bodies!

Studies link high cortisol levels to the development of insulin resistance and weight gain. So again, when we gain weight, our fat cells produce more estrogen. This results in estrogen dominance, mainly if our estrogen metabolism is not supported and healthy. So we have to take steps to lower our glucose and cortisol response.

Chapter 7

STRESSED TO THE MAX

Did you know that 75–90% of primary care visits are due to stress? When I saw this statistic, I was mind blown. If you think about it, though, who doesn't have stress?

Stress comes in many forms:

* Physical—from lack of sleep, illness, injury, physical exertion, extreme temperatures, or surgery.
* Metabolic—waste by-products from metabolism to normalize blood glucose, blood pressure and lipid levels.
* Emotional/Mental—worry, anxiety, depression, anger, over-thinking, relationship/marriage issues, lack of support, or pressure to meet deadlines.
* Chemical—from medications, toxins, heavy metals, and radiation.

SYMPATHETIC VS. PARASYMPATHETIC NERVOUS SYSTEM

When it comes to stress, it's essential to really understand the parasympathetic versus the sympathetic nervous system.

When your body is stressed, you move into fight or flight mode, also known as your sympathetic nervous system.

In this state, many body functions change, including:

* Increased heart rate and blood pressure

* Quick and shallow breathing
* Digestion and elimination stop
* Reproduction stops

If you're trying to conceive and your body is in a sympathetic state, your body doesn't even want to consider conception and pregnancy.

Remember, your body isn't meant to be in a constant sympathetic state. So when you are in that continuous or chronic sympathetic state, it starts to affect all your hormones and organs.

In a parasympathetic state, your:
* Heart rate slows down
* Blood pressure decreases
* Breathing becomes slow and deep
* Digestion and elimination occur normally
* Reproductive function resumes

If you want to be pregnant, your body is more ready for reproduction in a parasympathetic than in a sympathetic state.

Think of your uterus as the soil of a garden. You can take the proper nutrients to tend the soil. However, if the environment is hot, windy, and without rain, it creates a stressful environment. This will not bring nourishment to the seed and allow it to grow optimally or at all.

Now let's dive into how cortisol and sex hormones are made. I want you to better understand and appreciate why you need to get back to operating from primarily a parasympathetic state.

All your sex hormones and cortisol come from cholesterol but are produced in different areas of the body.

Adrenal glands:
* Cortisol
* DHEA
* Testosterone

Ovaries:
   * Testosterone
   * Estrogen
   * Progesterone

When your body is under stress, it will focus on sending signals from your brain to produce more cortisol. It is focused on protecting you. Remember: flight, fight, or freeze.

Usually, after a stressful event, cortisol does not stay elevated for long and comes back down. However, when you have back-to-back stressors, your adrenals keep releasing more cortisol. This causes a constant state of high cortisol.

When your brain signals your adrenals to produce more cortisol, it does not create more sex hormones. This is especially true of progesterone because your body will always choose survival over reproduction. Progesterone is the primary pregnancy hormone. When you are stressed, your body sends fewer signals to your ovaries to produce progesterone. In this way, stress results in low progesterone levels and hormonal imbalance.

I commonly see many chronically stressed women have lower levels of progesterone. Remember the different estrogen dominance patterns? This is the cause of two types of estrogen dominance. There are low progesterone levels in ratio to either high or normal levels of estrogen in these types.

Lower levels of progesterone tend to cause anxiety, mood swings, sleep disturbances, and infertility. Then if there are normal or higher levels of estrogen circulating in your body, this creates an estrogen dominance effect.

Chapter 8

ESTROGEN'S IMPACT ON YOUR THYROID

Your thyroid is mainly responsible for metabolism at a cellular level. It helps your cells:
   * Produce and store energy
   * Regulate heart rate and body temperature
   * Develop your brain
   * Build up or break down your bones

Your thyroid produces two hormones T4 and T3. Thyroid hormones comprise one tyrosine molecule, an amino acid, and either three iodine (T3) or four iodine (T4) molecules.

Iodine is not made in your body, so it must be consumed through food such as seaweed and shellfish. T4 converts a little into T3 in the thyroid. This conversion mainly occurs in your liver and other organs such as your kidneys, nervous system, fat cells, and muscles.

Most people don't realize that T3 is the most active thyroid hormone in the body. It's the hormone that is most often overlooked. Just checking TSH and T4 does not give us an overall view of how thyroid hormones are functioning in your body. There are even some people who are not able to convert T4 into T3 efficiently.

Many factors affect this conversion, such as:
   * Nutritional deficiencies
   * Food sensitivities
   * Poor gut health
   * Stress
   * Hormonal imbalance
   * Toxins

You need to address all these factors for optimal thyroid hormone function.

Another hormone called Thyroid Stimulating Hormone (TSH) is made and released from your pituitary gland. It helps regulate your thyroid to produce more thyroid hormones if levels are low.

Hypothyroidism occurs when your pituitary releases high levels of TSH, but your thyroid doesn't respond to this hormone to create more thyroid hormones. Usually, this is detected through blood work. We see high levels of TSH and low levels of T4 and T3.

Some people can develop subclinical hypothyroidism, which means they have symptoms of low thyroid function, but their levels are "within range." This can occur when TSH is on the upper end, and T4 and T3 are on the lower end of the normal range.

Hashimoto's is the autoimmune form of hypothyroidism. It occurs when there is an increase in thyroid antibodies such as Thyroid Peroxidase (TPO) antibody and Thyroglobulin Antibody.

Symptoms of hypothyroidism can include:
* Weight gain
* Scalp hair loss
* Loss of outer one-third of eyebrows
* Slow heart rate
* High cholesterol
* Fatigue
* Brain fog
* Dry skin
* Brittle/breaking nails
* Constipation
* Enlarged thyroid gland
* Sensitivity to cold

Hyperthyroidism is the opposite. Too much thyroid hormone is produced, and signals travel from the thyroid back to the pituitary gland. These signals tell the pituitary gland not to release more TSH. As a result, thyroid hormones are really high, and TSH levels are super low.

Grave's disease is the autoimmune disorder of hyperthyroidism. Lab values show elevated TPO, but more commonly, the elevation of Thyroid Stimulating Immunoglobulin (TSI).

Symptoms of hyperthyroidism include:
* Weight loss/inability to gain weight
* Mood swings
* Anxiety
* Rapid heart rate
* Hyperactivity
* Muscle weakness
* Diarrhea
* Trouble sleeping
* Bulging/puffy eyes
* Sensitivity to heat

Studies show that excess estrogen increases a protein that binds up thyroid hormones, especially T4 over T3, called Thyroid-Binding Globulin (TBG). When this happens, TSH increases due to low levels of T4. If your thyroid is not able to produce more thyroid hormone, then hypothyroidism occurs.

Excess estrogen is linked to increased inflammation in the body, especially in women with PCOS and Endometriosis. In turn, inflammation increases thyroid antibodies such as TPO and Thyroglobulin Antibody leading to Hashimoto's Thyroiditis.

These are the thyroid labs your practitioner should be checking:
* TSH
* Total T4
* Free T4
* Total T3
* Free T3
* Reverse T3
* For hypothyroid symptoms: TPO and thyroglobulin antibodies
* For hyperthyroid symptoms: TSI, TRAb and TPO

Chapter 9

IS HISTAMINE INTOLERANCE TO BLAME?

Histamine is a compound released from basophils and mast cells, which are part of your immune system. It's also released from gastric cells in your stomach that secrete stomach acid.

Histamine causes:
* Smooth muscle contraction
* Inflammation
* Dilation of blood vessels
* Releases cytokines (small proteins that are messengers of the immune system to increase or decrease inflammation)

Histamine also acts as a neurotransmitter in the brain to keep you awake. However, excess amounts are linked to the formation of addictive behaviors and neurodegenerative diseases such as Parkinson's and Multiple Sclerosis.

Histamine Intolerance occurs when there is an increase in the amount of histamine in your body that isn't broken down quickly.

Common causes of histamine intolerance include:
* Genetics
* Exposure to certain foods
* Chemicals
* Toxins
* Environmental (pollen, dust mites) allergens
* Microorganisms such as mold
* Overgrowth of bacteria in the small intestines (SIBO).

There is an enzyme called Diamine Oxidase (DAO) responsible for histamine breakdown in your body. However, some people have a genetic mutation of the DAO enzyme. This slows the function of DAO, preventing histamine from breaking down.

If you want to learn more about this enzyme and find out if you have this genetic mutation, I recommend reading Dr. Ben Lynch's book called "*Dirty Genes*" and doing his StrateGene test. For more information, check out the resources section at the end of this book.

Even though histamine intolerance is an immune response similar to an allergic reaction, it is different from acute allergies.

An acute allergic response occurs within minutes to an hour after exposure to an allergen. It causes symptoms of hives, swelling, or life-threatening anaphylaxis.

Histamine intolerance is more of a delayed response that occurs from the accumulation of histamines in the body.

Symptoms of Histamine Intolerance include similar symptoms as acute allergies, but so many more unexplainable symptoms such as:
* Headaches/Migraines
* Sinus congestion
* Runny nose
* Seasonal allergies
* Hives
* Eczema
* Rapid Heart Rate
* Low blood Pressure
* Asthma
* Bloating
* Diarrhea
* Nausea/vomiting
* Heartburn
* Abdominal Pain
* Menstrual Cramping/PMS
* Anxiety
* Irritability

Estrogen dominance contributes to the release of histamine from mast cells found in your reproductive organs. This occurs because estrogen and histamine attach to the same receptors, H1.

Higher amounts of histamine also contribute to excess estrogen release. This adds fuel to the fire and becomes a vicious cycle in your body.

If you suspect histamines are playing a role, the good news is that you can do something about it! This will result in significant improvement in your symptoms.

The first step is to remove foods high in histamine, foods that release histamine, and foods that block the DAO enzyme.

If you're not sure where to start or what to eat on a low histamine diet, I highly recommend checking out Dr. Becky Campbell's book "*The 4-Phase Histamine Reset Plan*." You can find this book on Amazon.

You can also take a DAO supplement sold by Seeking Health. I recommend having genetic testing before starting this supplement.

Some natural supplements that lower the histamine response in your body include:
* Quercetin
* Stinging Nettle
* Vitamin C

›› *Note: Take Quercetin with caution or avoid it if you have a sulfur allergy causing anaphylaxis, as it does contain a sulfur amino acid.*

Also, do not rely on supplements alone. You have to remove histamine foods and find other sources of allergens such as mold, SIBO, chemicals in your environment, etc. Histamine levels will remain elevated until the source is removed.

Chapter 10

HORMONAL CONDITIONS
CAUSED BY ESTROGEN DOMINANCE

ENDOMETRIOSIS

According to the World Health Organization, endometriosis is an estrogen-dominant condition that affects approximately 10%, about 190 million women. About 20–25% of those women don't know they have it. In fact, it can take about 7.5 years to get diagnosed.

What exactly is endometriosis?

It is a disorder where the lining of the uterus, called the endometrium, grows outside the uterus. This tissue becomes swollen and bleeds, causing pain and inflammation. It also causes scarring (called adhesions) inside the abdominal cavity or around the intestines and organs.

Endometrial tissue can be found around the ovaries, fallopian tubes, intestines, and the bladder.

When an imbalance of estrogen to progesterone exists, high levels of estrogen cause endometrial tissue to grow.

Symptoms of endometriosis include:
* Debilitating cramps
* Painful periods
* Pelvic pain
* Pain with bowel movements
* Painful sex
* Heavy bleeding
* Bleeding between periods
* Abdominal bloating

* Constipation
* Infertility

The most common conventional treatment is NSAIDs (ex. Motrin or Ibuprofen), birth control, and surgery. However, these treatments do not address the root cause, which is inflammation and an imbalance of the estrogen and progesterone ratio.

Adenomyosis occurs when the endometrium grows in the muscle wall of the uterus. This too, is from an imbalance of estrogen to progesterone, causing estrogen to thicken the endometrium.

Symptoms of adenomyosis include:
* Heavy, prolonged periods
* Blood clots
* Bleeding between periods
* Debilitating menstrual cramps
* Pelvic pain
* Painful sex
* Bloating

Like endometriosis, the conventional treatment can include taking birth control, NSAIDs for pain, or having a hysterectomy, which removes the uterus. But again, these treatments do not address the root cause.

POLYCYSTIC OVARIAN SYNDROME

Polycystic Ovarian Syndrome (PCOS) is another common disorder involving metabolic and hormonal imbalance. It is caused by insulin resistance and excess androgens, such as testosterone and DHEA.

High levels of insulin send signals to the ovaries to produce more testosterone. When there are too many androgens in the body, females take on male-like characteristics. These include excessive hair growth on the chin, chest, around the areolas, back, below the belly button, and buttocks.

Other symptoms include:
- Irregular periods, heavy periods
- Severe cramping
- Infertility
- Acne
- Oily skin
- Scalp hair loss
- Weight gain
- Blood sugar dysregulation contributing to insulin resistance and diabetes

PCOS causes some women to develop cysts on their ovaries and may even have ruptured cysts, causing abdominal pain. Cysts form when too much insulin causes the pituitary gland to release more LH than FSH.

If there is not enough FSH, the follicles cannot mature and the dominant follicle cannot form during ovulation. This delays or prevents ovulation causing irregular or no periods.

Ovarian cysts are not a required sign to receive a PCOS diagnosis. Some women with PCOS may not have ovarian cysts or weight gain. However, they may have many symptoms and signs through blood work that are consistent with the diagnosis. Unfortunately, medical professionals may dismiss them as not having PCOS because they don't have all the symptoms or signs.

The conventional treatment for PCOS is also NSAIDs and birth control. In addition, they're often prescribed androgen blockers, such as Spironolactone, and Metformin to stabilize glucose. However, these treatments only target the symptoms. They do not address the root cause.

Most importantly, studies show that women with PCOS have elevated androgens AND estrogens. This is important because if the estrogen levels are not addressed, then symptoms continue. After all, most of the symptoms of PCOS are also the same symptoms as estrogen dominance.

SHORT LUTEAL PHASE

The last hormonal imbalance I want to cover is Short Luteal Phase (aka Short Luteal Defect).

For an average 28 day cycle, the luteal phase lasts 14 days. However, as you know by now, it's normal for cycle length to vary by a couple of days either way. So if your luteal phase is less than 10 days, you have a short luteal phase.

Symptoms of Short Luteal Phase include:
- Frequent periods (having two every month)
- Spotting between periods
- Miscarriages
- Difficulty trying to conceive

Studies show that women with a cycle shorter than 26 days have higher estrogen levels in the follicular phase. This is the phase right before ovulation occurs. These women also had lower levels of progesterone in the luteal phase.

Remember, if estrogen levels are high and progesterone levels are low, this is one of the patterns of estrogen dominance. In fact, some of the causes of a short luteal phase are endometriosis and PCOS.

For optimal ranges of progesterone, testosterone, DHEA, and insulin check out the resources section at the end of this book.

Chapter 11

ESTROGEN'S ROLE IN
YOUR FERTILITY JOURNEY

According to the Centers for Disease and Control, about 10% of American women, about 6.1 million, have trouble getting pregnant or staying pregnant. Because of this, more and more women use assisted reproductive technology. The most common form is in-vitro fertilization (IVF). Approximately 1.9 million babies in the United States are born via these methods.

So why are women having trouble conceiving or maintaining pregnancy?

I believe that estrogen dominance is playing a huge role. But, unfortunately, it is overlooked as a possible root cause of infertility.

ESTROGEN AS BIRTH CONTROL

Remember, excess estrogen in the body acts like birth control. When progesterone is low during the luteal phase, this creates an estrogen dominant effect. Progesterone levels are not able to rise.

Progesterone is needed to change the uterine lining to prepare for implantation of the fertilized egg. If this does not happen, pregnancy does not occur.

I have already covered how stress can cause low progesterone levels. Nutritional deficiencies is another cause that gets overlooked. I will review nutritional supplements for progesterone support in Chapter 19.

PROGESTERONE RESISTANCE

Another way infertility occurs is from progesterone resistance. This occurs in endometriosis and PCOS when there is a disruption in the balance between progesterone and estrogen.

Yes, progesterone resistance is a thing.

This means that the uterus tissue does not respond to progesterone because of the excess amount of estrogen.

Normally the endometrium changes at a cellular level to get prepared for implantation of the fertilized egg. This occurs in the ovulatory phase of the menstrual cycle and is called endometrial decidualization. Estrogen dominance and progesterone resistance prevent the endometrium from changing at a cellular level.

INFLAMMATION & MICROTRAUMA

Studies also show that women with endometriosis and adenomyosis experience infertility due to the effects of extra estrogen on the uterus. This results in hyperperistalsis, a fancy medical term for increased contraction of the uterus during the menstrual cycle.

When this occurs, estrogen increases the production of prostaglandins. Prostaglandins are compounds that increase inflammation in the uterus. Increased contraction of the uterus leads to straining and microtrauma of the muscles and endometrium.

In addition to inflammation, the changes of the endometrium from microtrauma can prevent implantation from occurring.

SHORT LUTEAL PHASE

Lastly, when the luteal phase is less than 10 days, women may have issues with fertility. Normally progesterone, the pregnancy hormone, increases and reaches its peak during the luteal phase. The increase in progesterone changes the uterine lining, so implantation of a fertilized egg can occur.

When the luteal phase is too short, this cannot happen. This is because progesterone levels need to rise for pregnancy to occur. Therefore women who have a short luteal phase, may have low progesterone levels that cannot increase to maintain and sustain a pregnancy.

Thus, low progesterone levels in ratio to estrogen creates estrogen dominance.

Chapter 12

THE CONNECTION BETWEEN AUTOIMMUNE & ESTROGEN DOMINANCE

An autoimmune disorder occurs when high levels of antibodies start attacking your body's own cells.

Autoimmune disorders occur because of three things:
* Increased intestinal permeability (leaky gut)
* A triggering event (such as an inflammatory food, infection, trauma, or stress)
* Genetics

Approximately 80% of people with autoimmune disorders are women. So why do women have a higher risk of developing autoimmune diseases than men?

Studies reveal this is because women have two XX chromosomes. The X chromosome contains more genes than the Y chromosome (men have one X and are XY) and more genes that regulate the immune system.

Studies show that estrogen receptors are found not just in the breast, uterus, and ovaries. Instead, they are also all over the body in other organs such as the brain, thyroid, intestine, muscle, and bone.

Scientists discovered several key estrogen receptors, including Estrogen Receptor Alpha (ERα), Estrogen Receptor Beta (ERß), and G protein-coupled receptor (GPER1/GPR30).

These receptors regulate inflammation and the immune system. This also happens with too much estrogen, such as estrogen dominance, or too little, like during postmenopause.

For example, when estrogen binds more to ERß, this actually lowers inflammation and suppresses the growth of cells. Conversely, if more estrogen binds to ERα, it increases the growth of cells, inflammation and increases the immune system response.

Depending on their function, these estrogen receptors are either expressed or not expressed in those with autoimmune disorders. This leads to increased inflammation and upregulation of the immune system.

Another reason why women are more prone to developing autoimmune disorders is that we go through three transition periods throughout our lifetime. These transition phases cause a change in the levels of our hormones. They include puberty, pregnancy, and menopause.

Once women go through puberty, they produce higher levels of progesterone and estrogen, especially E1 and E2. Suppose these women have estrogen dominance and an autoimmune disorder. In that case, they may notice their symptoms flare one to two weeks before their period. Flares occur because of imbalanced or higher levels of estrogen.

Some women with autoimmune disorders may notice improvements in the autoimmune symptoms or go into remission during pregnancy. Remission can happen with conditions like Multiple Sclerosis. They occur because progesterone levels increase, and the body produces more estriol or E3, which has anti-inflammatory properties.

However, other women with autoimmune conditions may flare due to the higher levels of estrogen, especially those with Systemic Lupus Erythematosus (SLE).

As women go through menopause, they may notice worsening of their symptoms. This occurs due to the declining levels of estrogen that send signals to increase inflammation and upregulate the immune system.

HASHIMOTO'S THYROIDITIS

Hashimoto's Thyroiditis is an autoimmune disorder where thyroid antibodies such as Thyroid Peroxidase (TPO) and Thyroglobulin Antibody destroy thyroid tissue. When this happens, your thyroid can't produce enough of the thyroid hormone, which results in an underactive thyroid.

We previously discovered that excess estrogen can increase inflammation. This leads to increased levels of TPO and increased production of Thyroid Binding Globulin in the liver (TBG), which binds up T4.

RHEUMATOID ARTHRITIS

If you have Rheumatoid Arthritis (RA), your immune system develops antibodies such as Rheumatoid Factor (RF) and anti-Cyclic citrullinated peptide (anti-CCP). These antibodies attack your body's joints resulting in pain, swelling, bone erosion, and deformity of the joint.

There is a solid genetic component linked with RA. Still, Lyme disease has been discovered as another root cause of the development of RA.

Interestingly enough, studies show increased estrogen, especially the metabolites 16a-OHE1 and 4-OHE1, in the joint fluid of people with Rheumatoid Arthritis. Researchers believe this stimulates the inflammatory process of this autoimmune disorder.

LUPUS

There are four types of Lupus, but I will focus on Systemic Lupus Erythematosus (SLE) because it is the most common type.

SLE affects multiple organs such as skin, lungs, kidneys, heart, brain, blood vessels, muscles, tendons, and joints. I don't want to get too nerdy over the immune system pathways. Yet, I want to give you a general understanding of why this is important and how estrogens play a role in SLE.

T-helper 1 (TH1) and T-helper 2 (TH2) are immune system cells that produce specific cytokines depending on the activated immune response.

TH1 is responsible for killing viruses and bacteria in your body and stimulating an immune response within your cells (cellular immune response). The role of TH2 is to produce antibodies and regulate allergic reactions. This promotes an immune response in your body fluids (humoral immune response).

Studies show increased expression of Estrogen Receptor alpha in those with SLE resulting in shifting the balance of TH1/TH2 to Th1<Th2.

Th2 produces many cytokines, such as interleukin-10 (IL-10) and interleukin-6 (IL-6). These cytokines produce higher anti-dsDNA antibodies found in those with SLE in response to higher estrogen levels.

Also, higher levels of the estrogen metabolite 16a-OHE1 than 2-OHE1 were noted in women with SLE, which increases proliferation of cells. Normally 16a-OHE1 usually should be low or not detected.

CROHN'S AND ULCERATIVE COLITIS

Crohn's and Ulcerative Colitis are two autoimmune disorders classified as two types of Inflammatory Bowel Disease (IBD). This is caused by inflammation and destruction of the gut lining, which is different from Irritable Bowel Syndrome (IBS).

These two autoimmune disorders of the gut occur from many different factors, such as:
   * Genetics
   * Poor gut health from leaky gut and dysbiosis
   * Inflammatory foods

* Stress
* Increased immune responses

Studies show that the estrogen receptors alpha and beta, ERα and ERβ, also regulate inflammation and the immune system in the gut. The role of ERβ is to reduce inflammation and prevent the growth of cancerous cells. There are more ERβ in the intestines.

An increase in an immune-inflammatory cytokine called interleukin-6 (IL-6) causes a decrease in ERβ, which leads to inflammation in your intestines. It also causes upregulation of your immune system and can even increase your risk of colon cancer.

Chapter 13

THE TRUTH BEHIND BREAST IMPLANT ILLNESS AND BREAST CANCER

BREAST IMPLANT ILLNESS

About 400,000 women get breast implants every year. There are two common types of breast implants used today. Both have a silicone capsule and are filled with either saline or silicone.

Breast implants are deemed safe by the FDA. What they don't tell you is that they are not meant to last long term. They start breaking down in your body, including the silicone capsule.

All implants come with an expiration date and are not meant to be in your body past that time. Breast implants are foreign bodies. When there is a foreign body, your body will do everything in its power to attack it and get rid of it. Your body recognizes that it should not be there. This can increase your immune response and can be masked as an autoimmune disorder, chronic disease or infection.

Breast Implant Illness (BII) is a term to describe an inflammatory and immune response in the body that occurs from breast implants. It results in many different unexplainable symptoms after having breast implants placed.

Even though it is not a medical term, nor does it have its own diagnosis code, I believe it falls under the umbrella of Autoimmune/inflammatory Syndrome of Induced Adjuvants (ASIA).

In fact, some women develop other autoimmune disorders such as Hashimoto's, Sjogren's, Lupus, Rheumatoid arthritis, anywhere from a couple of months to a couple of years after getting breast implants. This could be from the increased immune and inflammatory response that occurs from having a foreign implant.

Common symptoms reported from those with suspected BII include:
* Fatigue
* Brain Fog
* Muscle or joint pain (generalized or specific to shoulder/arm/back)
* Anxiety or Depression
* Insomnia
* Shortness of Breath
* Skin rashes
* Dry eyes/mouth
* Gut issues
* Food sensitivities
* Low Libido
* Infertility

Many more symptoms have been reported, but these are the common ones. More symptoms reported can be found on: www.breastimplantillness.com

There are no tests to prove someone has breast implant illness, but we can access the body's systems for imbalances. Standard systems to check include:
* Gut
* Adrenals
* Sex hormones
* Detoxification
* Immune system
* Inflammatory markers

Breast implants also contain many chemicals. Heavy metals such as mercury, lead, arsenic, and platinum leak out of the silicone capsules. In fact, these heavy metals can bind to your estrogen receptors and disrupt your hormones resulting in irregular cycles and painful periods.

Even silicone itself diffuses through these capsules, called gel bleed. It deposits into surrounding tissue such as the lymph nodes and has been detected in the spinal cord and brain. These toxins are stored in the fat cells and affect liver detoxification. These chemicals are also known as xenoestrogens, which I'll discuss in Part III, which contribute to estrogen dominance.

BREAST CANCER

Did you know that only 9–10% of women that get breast cancer have the BRCA1 and/or BRCA2 gene?

So if only 9–10% of breast cancer patients have the BRCA1 and/or BRCA2 gene, what about the other 90%?

I believe it occurs from epigenetics, the lifestyle and environmental factors that affect our genes and metabolism at a cellular level.

Most of these women likely have other genetic mutations such as the COMT and MTHFR genes that affect estrogen metabolism and higher levels of 16a-OHE1 and 4-OHE1 that are not getting tested and addressed.

Studies show that women who have lower 2-OHE1 and 2/16-OHE1 ratios have a higher risk for breast cancer.

Remember, the estrogen metabolites 16a-OHE1 increase the growth of cancer cells, and 4-OHE1 damages DNA. Therefore having higher levels of both with lower levels of 2-OHE1 and 2-oMeE1 increases the risk of breast cancer.

How many women can prevent and reduce their risk by supporting the right metabolites and lowering the harmful ones? What if they also addressed lifestyle and environmental factors? This is why I want to bring awareness to educate and inspire more women to be more proactive in preventing breast cancer.

It is essential to understand the mechanism behind cancerous cell growth. In your breast, remember there are two receptors Estrogen Receptor Alpha (ERα) and Estrogen Receptor Beta (ERβ). These receptors have two functions.

When estrogen binds more to ERβ, it helps to suppress tumor growth. If more estrogen binds to ERα, it increases the proliferation of your breast cells, increasing tumor growth and leading to breast cancer.

Approximately 75% of breast cancer is ERα positive. Remember, there are estrogen receptors all over your body, including the uterus, thyroid, and lungs. Therefore, increased estrogen receptor expression that stimulates growth in other organs can also lead to cancer, not just in the breasts.

Studies show the link between increased expression of the estrogen receptors from excess estrogen to the development of thyroid, uterine, endometrial, colon, and metastatic bone cancer.

Does Soy or Flax Cause Breast Cancer?

Phytoestrogens are estrogen-like compounds found in plant foods. These include soy and flax, and they have weak estrogen activity. Because of this, breast cancer patients are told to avoid foods with these phytoestrogens, such as soy and flax.

Studies show that consuming flax and soy actually lowers your risk of breast cancer. In addition, even though phytoestrogens have weak estrogen effects, studies show they prefer to bind to ERβ, which helps reduce tumor growth!

In fact, when comparing American women to Asian women who consume more soy, Asian women have a one-third reduction in breast cancer risk. So therefore, I believe that the type of soy consumed could also play a role.

With the massive movement in 2018 towards veganism, more companies are making plant-based dairy and meat alternatives. One popular alternative is soy products ranging from soy milk, cheese, yogurt, and soy protein isolate.

However, these products, along with hydrogenated soybean oil, are all inflammatory forms of soy. If you choose plant-based options, avoid these types of soy!

You can consume soy to get the benefits such as isoflavones to fight against free radicals and reduce cancer risk. Just make sure it's as close to its natural form as possible and is organic and non-GMO, such as edamame and tempeh.

Even though tofu is "processed" soybeans to form a solid block, it is better than the other processed forms.

Other lifestyle factors contribute to an increased risk of breast cancer. For example, the food we consume, such as red meat and alcohol, is linked to an increased risk. Hormones from meat are xenoestrogens, and alcohol affects estrogen metabolism, which I'll talk about in the next chapter.

As I previously discussed, women who gain weight have higher estrogen levels produced from the fat tissue. In addition, studies show a link to women who are overweight or obese with an increased risk of breast cancer.

Other risk factors include women with a sedentary lifestyle and/or smokers.

Causes of Breast Cancer:
* Standard American Diet: High animal protein, refined carbs, sugar, and unhealthy fats
* Red Meat
* Alcohol
* Overweight/Obesity
* Sedentary Lifestyle
* Smoking

I hope we continue to learn more about our bodies at a cellular level. This helps not only improve our lifestyle and environmental factors but also supports the metabolization of estrogens. Improving estrogen metabolism can significantly reduce the amount of breast cancer that occurs.

Part III

MAKING HEALTHIER CHOICES
FOR HEALTHIER HORMONES

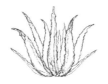

Chapter 14

TOXINS THAT MIMIC ESTROGEN

XENOESTROGENS

Xenoestrogens, aka endocrine disruptors, are foreign compounds from outside the body. They imitate estrogen within the body and bind to the same receptors as estrogen.

These compounds can be synthetic or natural. The natural xenoestrogens are called phytoestrogens. They are found in our food, and I referenced this in the Breast Cancer section.

Synthetic xenoestrogens are not natural sources. They are found in our environment and also in our food. Examples include:
* Plastic packaging of food and beverages
* Chemicals used in our home and on our bodies
* Non-stick coating on cookware
* Hormones added to animal products such as meat and dairy
* Industrial chemicals from paints
* Flame-retardants
* Adhesives
* Fiberglass
* Jet fuel
* Exhaust emissions from vehicles
* And so many more!

Most importantly, they are also found in products that women use every month... tampons and pads!

Because of the thinner cell walls of the vaginal canal, chemicals are more easily absorbed than the outer skin. So make sure what you are using vaginally is as clean as possible!

Here are 10 common chemicals that are xenoestrogens, or endocrine disruptors, that are found in your home.

Bisphenol A or BPA is a chemical discovered in plastics such as plastic water bottles, plastic food storage containers, and wrapping.

Parabens are found in artificial preservatives, cosmetic, and body care products. They are added to increase the shelf life by preventing and reducing the growth of bacteria and mold.

Phthalates are chemicals added to plastics to make them more soft and flexible and lubricants as a softener. Therefore, they can be found in personal care products such as nail polish, soap, shampoo, and hair spray. However, a study discovered that they are also found in period pads!

Per-and Polyfluoroalkyl substances, or PFAS, according to the EPA, are man-made chemicals found in many products such as food packaging, non-stick cookware, and stain and water repellent fabrics and carpet cleaners.

Polybrominated Diphenyl Ethers, aka PBDE, are flame-retardant chemicals found in furniture in your home such as your couch, mattress, rugs, curtains, or furniture padding, as well as paints, plastics, electronics such as TVs, and wire insulation.

Polychlorinated Biphenyl (PCBs) are mainly found in your home if you have fluorescent lighting fixtures, cable & wire insulators, thermal insulation such as fiberglass, used adhesives or tape, caulking to seal baseboards, or have used chemicals to finish your wood floor.

Triclosan is a common ingredient with antibacterial properties found in hand soap, body washes, toothpaste, and even food packaging.

Dioxin has been classified as likely to be carcinogenic by the EPA. It has been found in trace amounts in certain cosmetics and even tampons! It forms as a byproduct during the manufacturing process of some cosmetic ingredients or as a byproduct of the bleaching process for tampons. Also, suppose you see personal care products like shampoo, body washes, hand soaps that say they are SLS free, which is Sodium laureth or lauryl sulfate. In that case, that's because SLS contains traces of dioxin.

Atrazine is one of the most widely used herbicides in the US. If you are not using it in your yard but live in a community that maintains your yard, you may be exposed to this chemical. This, too is an endocrine disruptor.

Volatile Organic Compounds (VOC) are gasses that enter the air from vehicles, paints, pesticides, household cleaning supplies, glues & adhesives used for arts & crafts, permanent markers, copiers, printers, and even nail polish remover. The same study that discovered phthalates in period pads also found VOCs.

You've now learned about the different hormone disrupting chemicals that could be in your home. As a result, you may be thinking you need to live in a bubble to prevent exposure.

Don't worry! Obviously, this is not practical! You probably already know that it is impossible to entirely avoid all chemical exposure. This is why it is crucial to be aware of the chemicals in your home and environment. Then, you can take steps to reduce your exposures and help support your body's natural ability to detox.

I highly recommend checking out the Environmental Working Group's (EWG) Skin Deep Database. Download the Think Dirty app to see the toxic or "dirty" products in your home. The app will also help you to find less harmful, healthier products as replacements.

Thankfully, we now have many options for non-toxic period products. If you haven't yet, please switch out your pads and tampons! Check out the Resources section at the end of this book for products I recommend in your home, for your body, and your period.

Chapter 15

YOU REALLY ARE WHAT YOU EAT

Nutrition plays a vital role in supporting healthy hormones and estrogen metabolism. Unfortunately, the Standard American Diet (SAD) is high in animal protein, refined carbohydrates, sugar, and unhealthy fats. It's also low in fiber, nutrients, antioxidants, and healthy fats. This negatively impacts your hormones and estrogen metabolism.

In fact, studies show that when women consume higher-fat diets, they produce more bile to help break down those fats. In these cases, 40% of their calories come from fat. This includes animal fat (ex. red meat, bacon, cheese) and unhealthy fats (trans fats from fried and packaged foods).

Furthermore, women with these diets tend to have more gallbladder issues. This, in turn, affects gut health and estrogen metabolism.

Studies show higher estrogen levels, and higher breast cancer risk, in women who consume large amounts of animal products.

GUT AND HORMONE DISRUPTING FOODS

As you start your healthy hormone journey, it is important to be aware of the inflammatory foods that disrupt your gut and hormones.

The most inflammatory foods of the Standard American Diet are:
* Wheat
* Dairy
* Sugar
* Processed oils
* Red Meat

* Caffeine
* Alcohol

Wheat and dairy are two foods that people consume in large quantities. In the US, our food industry markets these foods as "healthy." However, these foods are not the same as they were many years ago, and the quality has decreased over time.

For example, wheat in the US contains more gluten than wheat in Europe and in other countries. The EWG detects glyphosate in many different wheat products, such as wheat pasta and cereal. Glyphosate is the chemical used in the popular weed killer called Round-Up.

Researchers are studying the link of glyphosate contributing to Celiac disease, which is a gluten allergy. It may even contribute to gluten sensitivity as well. I believe that most people have become sensitive or intolerant to gluten because of these two factors.

Many dairy products contain added hormones and antibiotics. These antibiotics kill off our gut microbiome, and added hormones only contribute to hormonal imbalances within our bodies.

Some people also react to different proteins in dairy, such as casein and whey. Others are lactose intolerant and respond negatively to sugar lactose. This is because their bodies have a decreased production of the enzyme lactase to break it down. Reacting to these proteins or lactose can then cause inflammation in your gut.

Gluten and dairy are the first items I recommend removing when healing the gut. Once your gut is healed, you can reintroduce these foods one at a time to see if there is a sensitivity or not. If you have a sensitivity, symptoms can occur within 72 hours of reintroduction. Some examples of symptoms you may experience with a food sensitivity include:
* Stomach ache
* Bloating
* Nausea
* Headache

* Sinus congestion
* Joint pain
* Rash
* Acne
* Fatigue

As I mentioned in Chapter 6, sugar is linked to insulin resistance, which impacts estrogen dominance. Most packaged food contains added sugar. Remember, women should only consume 24 grams or 6 teaspoons of sugar per day.

I recommend reading the labels and calculating how much sugar you are consuming daily. Added sugar is found in cereals, granola, snack bars, bread, jams, jellies, salad dressings, pasta sauces, crackers, chips, and ketchup, to name a few.

Yes, even chips!

I read a label to a client once for Lay's Baked chips, the third ingredient was corn starch which gets broken down into sugar, and the fourth was sugar.

I also recommend eliminating refined carbs such as white rice, bread, pasta, crackers, flour, and anything with "starch" in the ingredient list. These foods are broken down into sugar, cause inflammation in your gut, and disrupt your hormones.

Here is an example of how easy it is to consume more than 24 grams of sugar per day even when eating "healthy."

If you start your day with coffee and Natural Bliss (all-natural) Vanilla creamer, 1 tablespoon is 5 grams of sugar. But who measures out one tablespoon? Or do you pour it in until it turns the color you like? If so, it could add up to 10–15 grams or more.

Then you grab a banana with about 14 grams of sugar, and out the door you go. From just these two items, you're already met more than half your intake or your entire intake for the day.

For lunch, you have a sandwich with Canyon gluten-free bread which is 2 grams per slice from agave syrup and cane sugar. You fill your sandwich with preservative-free deli meat, lettuce, tomato, and cheese.

In the afternoon, you get the munchies, so you snack on a mixed berry Chobani flavored yogurt. Your snack has 17 grams of sugar.

You enjoy a healthy dinner with salmon, quinoa, and veggies. The total amount of sugar consumed is anywhere from 39–50 grams for the day!

See how easily it adds up?

Now I'm not saying all sugar is bad. You don't have to avoid everything with sugar, including fruit. However, it is important to be mindful of how much you consume each day.

You should also be aware of inflammatory oils. These include:
* Canola oil
* Vegetable oil
* Peanut oil
* Safflower oil
* Corn oil
* Hydrogenated palm oil
* Soybean oil

These all affect your gut health and your hormones. Each of these oils goes through refinement, bleaching, and deodorization (called RBD). Then, they are expeller pressed, meaning a machine is used to apply friction and pressure to squeeze the oil out of ground seeds. This process creates heat and can change the properties of the oil.

Hydrogenation occurs when hydrogen is added to the oil to make it more solid. This changes the structure of the fat in oils into trans fats. Studies show trans fats increase inflammation in your body.

Know that even healthy oils, such as olive and coconut, can go through RBD and can be expeller expressed! It's better to find and choose a cold-pressed and unrefined oil such as olive, avocado, coconut, and walnut oil.

You'd be amazed that so-called "healthy foods," such as vegetable chips, can actually contain inflammatory oils. For example, when you look at the label of Terra Chips, they use canola and safflower oil, which is another reason to read the labels. You don't need to be a nutritionist to read a label. Just know what to look for!

Alcohol and caffeine are two beverages metabolized through your liver. They impact estrogen metabolism by preventing the active forms of estrogen from being metabolized into their inactive state. This prevents excess estrogen from being eliminated in your poop.

Alcohol also depletes glutathione which is the most powerful antioxidant produced by your liver. It is essential for detoxification of chemicals and toxins and fighting against free radicals that can cause cancer.

Just one serving of alcohol depletes your glutathione! So it's definitely something to think about when you enjoy a serving or more.

Caffeine also stimulates your adrenal glands. This is also important to be mindful of, especially if you are stressed and have any adrenal dysfunction. Even though it gives you an energy boost, it can actually add to your problem.

Lastly, remember that red meat and poultry, such as chicken and turkey, can contain antibiotics and hormones. These chemicals are added to fight off infection and help the animals grow because of the demand for meat in this country.

Like dairy, when we ingest meat that contains added hormones and antibiotics, it disrupts your microbiome and increases hormone levels. Grass-fed, organic, cage-free animals do not have these chemicals. However, we don't know the quality of grass that the cows are eating. It could be contaminated with glyphosate, or other weed killers, insecticides, and fertilizers which also disrupt your hormones.

Chickens may also be fed corn or soy, which is usually genetically modified and inflammatory to their bodies. So if you do consume poultry, make sure they are fed organic grain and are not pumped with hormones and antibiotics.

So what should you focus on eating more of?

Studies show that women who eat more of a vegetarian and high fiber diet have increased elimination and lower circulating levels of estrogen. These diets are high in:

* Vegetables
* Fruits
* Nuts
* Seeds
* Whole grains

In addition to fiber, plant foods also contain more vitamins, minerals, healthy fats, and antioxidants than animal meat and processed, packaged food. This is why I believe in consuming a primarily plant-based diet primarily to support healthy hormones and estrogen metabolism.

But are you going to get enough protein?

This prevents many people from switching to a whole foods plant-based diet. The answer is yes! Protein exists in almost every plant food. Even a ¼ cup of broccoli contains 2.6 grams of protein.

Your body needs twenty amino acids to make protein to create our tissues and organs, hormones, enzymes, and neurotransmitters. Your body can make eleven of those on its own. The other nine must come from food.

I once learned in a nutrition class, that meat and eggs were the only food source that contains all nine essential amino acids. However, several plant sources have all of them, such as:

* Quinoa
* Soy

- Tempeh
- Hemp seeds
- Chia seeds
- Buckwheat
- Spirulina
- Moringa

For example, if you consume quinoa, black beans, hemp seeds, and vegetables in just one meal, you'll be getting at least 15–25 grams of protein. On average, people need about 0.8g/kg of protein per day. So if you are 120 lbs (120/2.2 = 54.5 kg), you would need about 44 grams of protein a day.

The recommended protein intake is 1.2g/kg, about 65 grams of protein per day for those who exercise and are active regularly. Adding in a plant based protein shake, like my favorite from Vivo Life, is an easy way to get an additional 20–25 grams.

If you wish to consume non-plant-based protein sources, I recommend wild caught fish that are low in mercury. High levels of mercury in the body can affect your gut, brain, nervous system, liver, metabolic pathways and contribute to estrogen dominance by binding to estrogen receptors.

To make it easy to remember which fish are low in mercury, think of the acronym SMASH, which is salmon, mackerel, anchovy, sardines, and herring. I also recommend wild caught because it is caught in its natural habitat. In addition, it isn't farm raised, which tends to be high in antibiotics and hormones.

At the end of this book, I will provide a 28 Day plan which supports a plant-centered meal plan. It is also essential to substitute inflammatory foods for anti-inflammatory, nutrient-dense food and beverages.

Chapter 16

ADAPTING TO STRESS

I don't know about you, but I was never taught growing up how to manage stress. When I saw my primary care provider, I never mentioned I was stressed. However, they assumed that a lot of the symptoms I had, such as migraines and temporomandibular joint syndrome (TMJ), were from stress. Therefore, they would recommend antidepressants or anti-anxiety medications.

I finally gave in when I was in Physician Assistant school, because I had migraines every other day from the amount of stress I put on myself. What I discovered was that Prozac didn't get rid of the stress or my symptoms.

Instead, I felt numb and less in tune with my emotions. I realized this was not the state that I wanted to live my life, and I stopped taking it once I finished my clinical year.

However, the stress didn't disappear when I graduated and started working. Instead, it actually got worse. Eventually, I reached a point when I realized I needed to do something to control the anxiety I was experiencing. In addition, it affected my relationship with my husband. You see, we were in our first year of marriage. With the way it was going, we were headed for divorce.

From that point on, I was determined to work on my mindset. I discovered different ways to help my body adapt to stress, which was a game-changer for me! I will share these tips throughout the rest of this book, so stick around!

Please see your licensed medical provider if you are taking medications for stress, anxiety, or depression and want to stop. It is important that you do not quit cold turkey. Instead, you must be weaned off them to avoid severe side effects.

In the meantime, I will provide you with different ways to help you adapt to stress. I call them adaptation activities. They will help you to wean off and get you better results than taking medication.

ADAPTATION ACTIVITIES

Meditate

Many people have the misconception that meditation is sitting still with a blank mind devoid of all thoughts. However, you do not have to be a mini Buddha to meditate. Believe it or not, you have about 70,000 thoughts per day. Of these thoughts, 80% are negative, and 95% are repetitive from the day before.

Meditation is actually a great time to tune into your thoughts. You can notice and practice reframing your thoughts to more empowering ones that serve you better.

If you have never meditated, I recommend starting out by meditating for 5–10 minutes each day. There are many great books, programs, and apps for meditation which I have outlined in the resources section at the end of this book.

If you are used to meditating, I recommend at least 15–20 minutes a day. You can work up to two sessions a day. Studies show that meditation helps lower cortisol, as well as improve your mood and wellbeing. I definitely feel calmer and refreshed after meditating!

Yoga

Another great way to lower stress is by practicing yoga. Interestingly, studies back up its benefits.

Yoga lowers stress because it helps you connect back to your breath and puts you into a parasympathetic state. I also believe that stress or even trauma, whether physical or emotional, gets lodged into our tissues. I always find that yoga helps to release the tension in my body. I feel as if I have gotten a massage afterward because my muscles are so relaxed!

There are many different types of yoga, such as Vinyasa, Yin, Kundalini, Bikram, Hatha, Restorative, and Hot Yoga. If you're new to yoga, try popping into a local yoga studio for a sample class. You can also download an app with a guided yoga workout or find a yoga video on YouTube. This way you can try the different types and find the one that you enjoy most. I recommend doing at least 30–60 minutes of yoga 2–3 times a week.

Epsom Salt

Epsom salt baths are great to end the day and help your body to relax. Epsom salts are made from magnesium, sulfur, and oxygen. Magnesium is actually an anti-anxiety mineral that we need for many different metabolic processes. It also supports your adrenals, and it's a natural muscle relaxant.

You typically deplete magnesium when you are stressed. As a result, your body will further pull from your magnesium stores to:
* Make energy
* Build tissues
* Detoxify your cells

You also lose magnesium through sweat when you exercise. This is why many of us are actually deficient in magnesium. Epsom salts are one way to get some magnesium, but absorption through the skin is not enough. I recommend following up with a functional medicine practitioner to test your levels to determine if you need to take a supplement.

Belly breathing

Deep breathing, especially belly breathing or diaphragmatic breathing, is found to stimulate your Vagus nerve. This will slow down your heart rate and help your body to get back into a parasympathetic state.

Most of us breathe with our chest, so I recommend practicing more belly breathing. To do this:

* Sit comfortably with a hand over your belly.
* Inhale through your nose while expanding your belly and feel your stomach rise.
* As you exhale, relax your belly as the air flows out.

There are many deep breathing techniques such as the 4x4, 4–7–8, 4–2–6, and 2x breath (by Emily Fletcher). Try each one and see which one you like best. Try belly breathing for 5–10 minutes each day, especially when you feel any form of stress or tension in your body.

Creativity

Did you know coloring isn't just for kids? I personally love coloring and have found it helpful to reduce stress.

Journaling is also a great way to put thoughts onto paper. When you have many ideas or a list of things to do, writing them down can help reduce stress. It keeps your brain from constantly trying to remember and use energy to store this information.

Another way to get creative is to make or listen to music. Studies show that music helps to reduce anxiety and stress.

Grounding

Grounding or earthing is a beautiful way to help you reconnect and come in contact with the earth. It's a fancy name for walking barefoot or sitting on the earth.

The earth has natural electrical charges, called pulsed electromagnetic fields, or PEMF for short. PEMFs can stabilize your physiology to reduce stress, inflammation, improve the immune system, and promote wound healing. It's also used as a form of therapy for autoimmune disorders.

I recommend devoting at least 5–10 minutes outside daily if the weather permits. You can do this in your own yard if you have one, or go to a local park and sit on the grass, or go to the beach and walk barefoot in the sand.

Reframing

William Shakespeare once said, "There is nothing either good or bad, but thinking makes it so." Reframing is a great mindset tool that has been pivotal for me during stressful times of my life. Typically, I am stressed because of the perception and meaning I give to a person, place, event, or situation.

So next time you are stressed, take a step back and take a different perspective on what is causing the stress. For example, say to yourself, "Is there another way to look at this?" or "What story am I telling about this person, place, or situation, and is this story the truth?"

The mindset is very important to work on when it comes to stress and overall health. I believe that our cells hear our thoughts and have the power to create health or disease in the body.

After reading the different activities to help you adapt to stress, hopefully, there are 1–2 activities that stood out for you. I encourage you to make time in your day to do these activities. They can really make a difference in how you show up and the outcome of your day.

These activities have definitely been a game-changer for me. I no longer need or even think about taking medication to overcome stress.

Now let's get into the next lifestyle factor which is probably the most important of them all!

Chapter 17

SLEEP: THE MOST OVERLOOKED LIFESTYLE FACTOR

Are you falling asleep with ease and waking up feeling refreshed? If not, this means you're probably not getting good quality and quantity sleep.

Studies show that it is essential to get 7–8 hours of quality sleep per night for your overall health. It also helps to reduce the development of chronic disorders.

In fact, out of all the lifestyle factors, I believe that sleep is probably the most important one to focus on first. Without getting excellent quality and quantity sleep, it will impact every area in your life, including your energy, mood, and hormones. I say quality sleep because there are people who get 7–8 hours of sleep that still do not feel rested and restored. Their sleep is of poor quality.

Before I dive into what quality sleep is, let's review the benefits. The first benefit of sleep is that it reduces stress. I've already discussed how stress negatively impacts your hormones.

If you're not getting enough sleep, it creates inflammation in your body and raises cortisol levels. In turn, this causes low progesterone levels and creates an estrogen dominant state.

Insulin resistance commonly occurs from high levels of cortisol and estrogen. Sleep also lowers glucose levels which is important to prevent the development of insulin resistance.

Your body also repairs and restores its cells while you sleep. This is why you'll feel refreshed in the morning when you wake up if you get enough quality sleep. Quality sleep even helps support a healthy immune system.

Two other benefits of sleep are to improve your memory and mood. I can definitely focus better and have more clarity when I get 7–8 hours of quality sleep. So sleep is vital for brain health, and studies show that getting quality sleep lowers your risk of Alzheimer's disease.

Lastly, studies show that getting enough quality sleep helps to maintain a healthy weight. This is because lack of quality and quantity sleep decreases a hormone called Leptin. This hormone enables you to feel satisfied after eating.

Unfortunately, poor sleep also increases a hormone called Ghrelin which gives you the munchies. High levels of Ghrelin are linked to weight gain and obesity.

In fact, a study showed that a single night of sleep deprivation of about 4 hours resulted in an increase in Ghrelin and hunger. If you have the munchies at night, I suggest getting to bed earlier. Make sure you are getting 7–8 hours of quality sleep which will help you kick those cravings and promote a healthier weight.

Now let's focus on getting quality sleep which depends on the length of time spent in different stages of sleep. There are a total of four stages of sleep, but two of those stages impact the quality of your sleep.

Stage I: The first stage of sleep is when you start to fall asleep, known as light sleep.

Stage II: Once you start to fall asleep, you move into stage II of light sleep, where your heart rate slows down, and body temperature starts to drop.

Stage III: The next stage is stage III, which is called deep sleep. During this critical stage, your body repairs and restores its cells. Your brain flushes out toxins from metabolic waste. This is what I like to call cellular junk, because your brain has mitochondria that produce energy throughout the day. That process is called the glymphatic system. It is your brain's unique lymphatic system since it has a tight blood-brain barrier that prevents many things from passing through.

Have you ever felt hungover from not getting enough sleep? This is called brain fog and results from that cellular junk not getting removed while you sleep. Deep sleep accounts for about 20–25% of the total sleep, around 1.5 hours.

Stage IV: The last stage is REM, which is also known as rapid eye movement. During this stage, your heart rate and blood pressure increase. Dreaming occurs during REM sleep, as well as memory consolidation and creativity. This is also an important sleep stage, especially when storing memories and using our creativity. REM should also make up about 20–25% of total sleep and be around 1.5 hours.

We should be cycling through stages II, III, and IV throughout the night. When I previously learned about sleep, I thought we cycle through each stage like this: stage II › stage III › stage IV. However, when I started tracking my sleep, I discovered that I typically get more deep sleep (stage III) during the first half of my sleep. Then, I get more REM (stage IV) during the second half of my sleep.

So far, the best way to track the quality and quality of your sleep and learn your unique sleep patterns is using a wearable device such as an Oūra ring. There are other wearable devices out there in the form of a watch. What I like about the Oūra ring the best is that it has an airplane mode. As a result, it can reduce the Electromagnetic Fields (EMFs) emitted while I sleep, which I'll talk about next.

HOW DO YOU IMPROVE THE QUALITY AND QUANTITY OF SLEEP?

Sun Exposure

Our bodies follow a 24-hour circadian rhythm. Light suppresses melatonin levels during the day. Lack of light is what triggers your body to produce melatonin at night to induce sleep. Most of us work inside from sunup to sundown, so we don't get exposed to natural light. Our brain needs light to signal our 24-hour circadian rhythm. Getting daily sunlight exposure is a great way to improve sleep. Getting as little as 10–15 minutes of sunlight in the morning, even during a break, helps reset your circadian rhythm.

Orange Or Red Light

Dimming the lights in the evening when the sun goes down is a great way to signal your brain that it is time to wind down. I recommend buying Himalayan salt lamps or bulbs that have a red or a warm orange glow. This simulates the warm glow of the firelight that our ancestors had long ago before electricity.

At bedtime, cortisol levels should be at their lowest to allow melatonin levels to increase. However, if cortisol levels are higher at bedtime, this can create difficulty falling asleep. Most people will feel wired but tired when they have higher cortisol levels at bedtime.

There are many reasons why cortisol may be higher at bedtime. For example, bright lights send signals to your brain, making it think it is still daytime. This causes you to continue to produce cortisol.

Studies show that red or orange light helps your body produce more melatonin which you need to promote sleep. Higher cortisol levels are also due to:
* Not winding down before bedtime
* Exercising before bedtime
* Constantly worrying or thinking about all the things you have to do tomorrow or by a specific date.

Brain Dump

If you have many thoughts and to-do's running through your head, grab a journal and do a brain dump by writing it all down before you go to bed. Trust me, this works!

Reduce Emfs

Also, turning off all your electronics, including phones, laptops, computers, TVs, and routers, reduces EMF exposure (which is electromagnetic fields). Just like exposure to bright blue light from electronics, studies show the EMFs can negatively impact the quality of your sleep.

Sleep Schedule

Setting a sleep schedule can also improve your sleep. Typically people plan their day according to everything they have to do and sacrifice their sleep to get it all done. I don't know why we have adopted this mentality because lack of sleep affects our memory and performance.

I don't know about you, but I'd rather get great sleep and be productive for 3–4 hours than take 3–4 days to take care of things because I can't think and am exhausted.

Instead, focus on planning your day around your sleep. Sleep should be the first thing you prioritize, so make sure you set up a consistent sleep schedule to get 7–8 hours of sleep. Then you can plan your day once you figure out your sleep schedule.

Also, make a note of where you are spending a lot of your time. Most of us are addicted to our phones. I'll admit I get addicted too if I'm not mindful. It's easy to get caught up in scrolling on social media, which can waste a lot of time throughout the day. This time adds up and can be spent doing something more productive to improve your health or help you to grow!

You'll also want to make sure you are going to bed and waking up around the same time every day, as this helps to maintain a regular circadian rhythm. Once you wake up, don't hit snooze. When you hit snooze, it makes it harder to wake up. You may ruin your sleep cycle and wake up in the middle of REM which makes you feel more tired and groggy than refreshed even after 7–8 hours of sleep.

Caffeine & Alcohol

Avoiding alcohol, especially 5–6 hours before bedtime, can improve the quality of your sleep. Many people feel like alcohol helps them sleep. Unfortunately, this is only partially true. It may help you fall asleep, but then alcohol reduces the amount of REM sleep.

Also, don't drink caffeine any later than noon, especially if you are a poor caffeine metabolizer. Caffeine is a stimulant and takes about 5 hours for half the amount to break down.

For example, a cup of coffee has about 200mg of caffeine, so 5 hours later, there is still 100mg of caffeine in your system. By the time you're ready to wind down, you still have 100mg of caffeine circulating around!

Early Dinner

I also recommend eating your dinner earlier, or at least 3–4 hours before bedtime, because it takes about 3–4 hours to digest food. If you eat 1–2 hours before bed, you are still digesting and not resting.

I noticed this with myself once I started tracking my sleep. Eating close to my bedtime impacted my heart rate and heart rate variability, which determined how well I recovered during sleep.

I noticed my heart rate was higher, and my heart rate variability was lower when I ate even 1.5 hours before bed. Heart rate variability is the amount of time between your heartbeats. It assesses the sympathetic vs. parasympathetic response in your body to determine how well your body recovers during sleep.

There isn't an optimal range for heart rate variability, as this is different for each person. Still, you can track your own pattern with the Oūra ring.

Sleep Sanctuary

Lastly, I recommend creating a sleep sanctuary. You'll want to create a space that is clean, calm, and relaxing.

I don't know about you, but walking into a room with clothes lying everywhere, the sheets crumbed on the bed, and boxes stacked in a corner does not look like a sleep sanctuary to me!

My ideal sleep sanctuary has a bed with big fluffy pillows. The sheets are made from bamboo and are soft, cool, and breathable. I like duvet covers that make me feel like I'm sleeping on a cloud. My mattress is good quality, non-toxic (like Avocado), and I have a diffuser with essential oils. I have calming music playing and a Himalayan salt lamp emitting a nice warm glow.

Keep in mind that the temperature of your room will affect sleep quality as well. According to The Sleep Foundation, the recommended temperature is 60–67 degrees Fahrenheit. Suppose you implement all these steps and still aren't getting good quality or quantity sleep. In that case, I recommend following up with a Functional Medicine Practitioner to get checked out.

Chapter 18

EXERCISING FOR YOUR HORMONES

Believe it or not, exercise is crucial when it comes to your hormones and your overall health. Exercise is physical stress on your body, so keep in mind that the type of exercise you choose makes a difference.

If you currently have mental or emotional stressors, hormonal imbalances such as PCOS, adrenal, or immune disorders, then high-intensity exercise may not be the best type of exercise for you.

Many women engage in high-intensity exercise such as running marathons, going to CrossFit or Orange Theory, or doing High Intensity Interval Training (HIIT) workouts. I think that women who participate in these programs are amazing & inspiring! However, they have to be mindful of the impact those types of activities can have on their health.

Suppose you have adrenal dysfunction, hormonal imbalances, and/or have trouble losing weight or gaining weight. In that case, high-intensity exercise may be detrimental to your health and hormones.

It is essential to understand that during and after exercise, it is normal for cortisol to increase. Though, it should not remain elevated for long. When your body is under a lot of stress and put through high-intensity exercise, it causes even higher cortisol levels. In this case, they continue to stay elevated long term.

I'll go over the best exercises you can do that sync with your cycle and energy levels to support your hormones. But, first, let's review the fantastic benefits of exercise.

BENEFITS OF EXERCISE

Benefit #1: Lowers Glucose

The first benefit is that exercise helps to lower glucose. By doing so, it also improves insulin sensitivity. This one is a no-brainer because your body uses glucose as your first fuel source as you exercise. Therefore, if you have lower levels of glucose, you have better insulin sensitivity.

This means that your pancreas doesn't have to pump out a lot of insulin to lower glucose in your blood by driving it into cells for fuel or storage. Insulin resistance occurs when your cells do not respond to insulin, and glucose doesn't quickly enter your cells.

If this happens long-term, your pancreas can't keep up with the demand. It can also cause cellular damage to your pancreas. Such damage usually results in the development of Diabetes Mellitus Type II.

Estrogen dominance can create insulin resistance in your body, which also is an underlying cause of diabetes. However, studies show that a little bit of exercise such as a power walk or even yoga can help lower glucose levels after eating.

Benefit #2: Improved Mood And Memory

Ever seen the movie "Legally Blond?" In it, the very bubbly Reese Whitherspoon states, "Exercise gives you endorphins, and endorphins make you happy!"

Endorphins are hormones excreted in your brain and nervous system that are chemically similar to morphine. They give you the feeling of pleasure, reduce pain, and relieve stress.

Studies show that exercise also increases brain-derived neurotrophic factor (BDNF) that helps create new neural pathways in your brain associated with learning and memory.

In fact, higher levels of BNDF are associated with a lower risk of developing Alzheimer's and dementia. So if you want to learn a new skill or are reading something educational, get some exercise to strengthen those neural pathways!

Benefit #3: Improved Sleep

Exercise also improves the quality of your sleep. Studies show that 30 minutes of regular aerobic exercise can help you fall asleep faster and enhance deep sleep. However, it is best to exercise in the morning because if you exercise in the evening, it causes an increase in cortisol and body temperature. Both factors negatively impact your ability to fall asleep or get quality sleep.

Cortisol should be low at bedtime to allow melatonin levels to increase. If you are exercising before bed and having trouble falling asleep, this is because your cortisol levels are too high. High cortisol levels won't allow melatonin to increase.

Keep in mind that if you don't get quality sleep, you'll feel more tired overall. In addition, fatigue negatively impacts your physical performance and stamina when exercising.

Benefit #4: Better Energy

Another benefit of exercise is that it actually improves energy, just not when you are sleep-deprived. When you exercise, your muscles produce more mitochondria which are the powerhouse of your cells to help make energy.

So the more mitochondria your muscles have, the more energy your body can produce. I know I definitely feel more energy throughout the day after I exercise in the morning.

If you are not feeling energized throughout the day after you exercise, there is a possibility that you may have over-exerted yourself or you did not get quality sleep the night before. You may also have adrenal dysfunction or are not getting the proper nutrients to fuel your cells and help the mitochondria produce energy.

Benefit #5: Weight Management

In addition to getting great quality sleep, exercise also helps you maintain a healthy weight.

You must focus on all the lifestyle factors and not just one. Many factors play into your ability to lose weight. You can't expect to maintain a healthy weight if you're only focusing on just exercise and not improving the quality of your sleep, reducing stress, and eating whatever you want.

However, if you are doing all the lifestyle factors such as eating clean, whole foods, getting excellent quality and quantity sleep every night, exercising, doing adaptation activities, and you're still not able to lose weight, then it's time to check your gut and hormones for imbalances.

EXERCISING WITH YOUR CYCLE

Have you noticed there are times during your menstrual cycle that you do not feel motivated to exercise? This can be due to the fluctuation of your hormones.

During your period, it's normal to have lower energy levels and feel less active, especially if you have PMS symptoms. However, light exercise and low-impact activities can actually help improve menstrual cramps and mood.

Once you finish your period, your estrogen levels rise right before ovulation. As a result, you may gain more energy and physical stamina, which is better for aerobic or cardio exercise.

As you approach ovulation, you will feel your strongest and have the most energy. This is the best time to enjoy those higher intensity exercises.

However, if you have any type of adrenal dysfunction or hormonal imbalance, such as PCOS, these exercises might be best avoided.

After ovulation, you move into the luteal phase. At this point, you may find that your exercise tolerance and energy start to decline again. Your body temperature increases due to the rise in progesterone. Therefore, you are not able to cool down as effectively.

You definitely want to do low to moderate impact exercise to help your body recover during this time. I'll dive more into the specific types of activities for each cycle phase at the end of this book.

If you aren't currently exercising or don't know which exercises are best, I recommend creating an exercise routine that syncs with your cycle. But before you do, please check with your licensed medical provider before starting any exercise routine.

Chapter 19

YOUR GUIDE TO NATURAL REMEDIES AND SUPPLEMENTATION

Next, I want to dive into natural remedies and supplements that are helpful for hormonal balance.

I want to provide a disclaimer to make sure you understand that this information is for educational purposes only. Before taking any supplement or using any natural remedy, please consult with a licensed medical provider. This person should know your medical history. Do not take anything if you are pregnant without consulting with your provider first.

Another thing to remember is that not all supplements are created equal. Some may have blends or individual ingredients that are not at the proper dosage. Look at the "other" ingredients list on the label. They should not be a paragraph long and contain many added ingredients. These can include fillers, thickeners, dyes, and preservatives.

You'll want to find a reputable company that does third-party testing (because GNC or Walmart just doesn't cut it). The manufacturer should use pharmaceutical-grade ingredients, avoid allergens such as wheat, soy, dairy, etc. If possible, choose a supplement that is organic and non-GMO.

Also, keep in mind that these remedies may help relieve the symptoms but do not treat the root cause. Therefore, it is also essential to follow up with a certified Functional Medicine licensed medical practitioner or a Naturopath to get to the bottom of the problem.

Here are my favorite remedies for menstrual cramps, constipation, boating, and headaches.

MENSTRUAL CRAMP REMEDIES

Curcumin 1000–2000mg daily—Instead of taking Advil, Aleve, Motrin, etc., I recommend taking Curcumin. It is an antioxidant found in Turmeric, and it has anti-inflammatory properties.

We experience cramping because prostaglandins, which are hormone-like substances, are released to contract the uterus. It needs to contract to shed the endometrial lining, but it can result in pain and inflammation.

Curcumin can help reduce pain and inflammation naturally. However, it does not have immediate effects, so I recommend taking it 1–2 days before you know you are about to start your period.

Magnesium 200–400mg daily—Magnesium is a fantastic mineral that can relax your muscles and help ease cramps. In addition, when your uterus contracts to shed your endometrial lining, magnesium can help reduce the intensity of the contractions. In the supplements section, I'll dive more into the different types of magnesium.

Heating Pad—Whether it is electric or the old-fashioned rubber water type, a heating pad can also help relax your uterine muscles and reduce pain. However, I recommend using it only for 10–15 minute intervals because prolonged heat can also increase inflammation.

Essential Oils—Essential oils have excellent anti-inflammatory and muscle relaxing properties. These oils include lavender, frankincense, and peppermint oil.

You can apply these to the skin around the lower abdominal region where cramping occurs. However, make sure you dilute the oils with a carrier oil such as coconut, almond, or jojoba oil. Even one drop is concentrated and can irritate or burn the skin.

Red Raspberry Leaf—Lastly, red raspberry leaf has been used as a uterine tonic during menstruation and labor for at least two centuries.

This is because it actually has simulating and inhibitory effects, which help relax your uterus during menstruation.

In pregnancy, it can ease labor pains and help shorten labor. It has also been found to contain anti-inflammatory properties and many nutrients such as Vitamin A, C, E, calcium, iron, and potassium. You can find this in tea and tincture form. If you chose tea, drink 2–3 cups daily. I love drinking the tea, but the tincture is excellent for on the go!

›› *Precautions: Monitor your blood sugar as red raspberry leaf can lower blood glucose. It may also have weak estrogen effects, so it should be avoided in those with estrogen-positive breast, ovarian, and uterine cancer and used with caution in those with endometriosis and uterine fibroids.*

CONSTIPATION AND BLOATING REMEDIES

If you experience constipation and/or bloating, it's essential to see a functional medicine practitioner. You need to get your microbiome tested to determine the cause. Just treating the symptoms does not address the underlying problem. The issue can continue to worsen over time and result in more problems and imbalances in your body.

In the meantime, here are some remedies that can help improve your bowel movements. They can also help relieve bloating until the underlying cause is addressed.

Magnesium oxide 200–400mg—This form of magnesium helps to relieve constipation. It releases water into the stool to soften it and allow for easier passage.

Triphala 500mg daily—Triphala is a natural herb that helps promote bowel movements. However, if you are taking diabetic or high blood pressure medication, use caution. This herb could decrease the effectiveness of these medications causing glucose or blood pressure to increase.

Vitamin C 1000–2000mg daily—Vitamin C is a water-soluble vitamin. If you take high doses, you will reach "bowel tolerance" and experience a laxative effect. Plus, your body can only absorb 250–500mg at a time. So if you are taking more than that dose, your body gets rid of the rest.

Ground Flax or Psyllium Husk—Both are excellent sources of fiber which helps to absorb more water into the stool to add bulk, which allows for easier passage. I recommend taking 1 tablespoon of either in 8 ounces of water each morning.

If you opt for flaxseed, buy whole flaxseed and grind them fresh daily. This will allow you more nutrients than if you buy them pre-ground.

SIBO can worsen bloating and constipation with psyllium husk usage. If you experience worsening of your symptoms, see a Functional Medicine practitioner to get your gut checked.

Aloe Vera—Aloe has natural laxative properties and can help soothe the lining of your gut. You can buy fresh aloe at the store and add the gel to your smoothies or juice the aloe leaves. You can also purchase aloe juice and drink it daily.
>> *Precautions: Aloe can cause side effects such as diarrhea, abdominal cramps, dehydration, low blood sugar, and allergic reactions. If this occurs, stop drinking it immediately and do not continue to use it.*

It can react with certain medications such as Warfarin (Coumadin), Digoxin (for arrhythmias), and Diuretics (water pills such as Hydrochlorothiazide, Lasix, Spironolactone), and diabetic medications (such as Metformin, Glipizide, etc.).

Gaia Gas & Bloating—When I experienced severe bloating, this product helped relieve the bloat until I discovered the root cause and healed my gut. It contains activated charcoal and fennel that helps absorb gas and other calming herbs, such as chamomile, peppermint, licorice, and star anise. This comes in tea or capsules.

>> *Precautions: Because it has licorice, do not take this if you have high blood pressure. Also, note that sometimes charcoal can cause constipation or worsen constipation. Stop immediately if your symptoms increase.*

Probiotics—Probiotics are good bacteria that help to promote a healthy, robust microbiome. However, if you are constipated and possibly have SIBO, not all probiotics are helpful. Some can actually leave you feeling worse.

For example, Lactobacillus and Bifidobacteria are great probiotics that promote a healthy microbiome. However, some forms of SIBO are caused by both of these species of bacteria.

If you have histamine intolerance, you'll also want to avoid the mainstream probiotics because four strains of Lactobacillus release histamine in the gut. These include:
- Lactobacillus acidophilus
- Lactobacillus Casei
- Lactobacillus Bulgaria
- Lactobacillus Reuteri

Instead, I usually recommend starting with a spore-based probiotic, which is the Bacillus species that won't worsen the symptoms of SIBO. Consuming fermented foods can also help replenish gut bacteria. Again, if you have SIBO or histamine intolerance, this can worsen your symptoms.

HEADACHE REMEDIES

I suffered from migraines for many years until I got my body back into balance by healing the gut and rebalancing my hormones. When I would get them, I would take Tylenol, Advil, and prescription medications called Fioricet and Imitrex to treat them.

During my Functional Medicine certification, I discovered Advil disrupts the microbiome and gut lining, contributing to leaky gut. In addition, Tylenol depletes glutathione, so I chose to never take them again.

I found that there were natural remedies to treat headaches. The key was to be proactive as soon as I started to feel one coming on. Thankfully, I don't get them often anymore. But, if I do, I rely on these natural remedies.

Hydrate—First and foremost, most headaches and migraines occur from dehydration. So make sure you're drinking plenty of water daily, at least half of your body weight in ounces. If you start to feel a headache coming on, immediately increase your water intake. Sometimes that is all your body needs, and if it is, it should subside shortly after hydrating.

Magnesium 200–400mg—Take magnesium daily, which has been shown to help reduce the frequency or even prevent migraines. You can also take an Epsom salt bath with magnesium salts to help relax the muscles at the onset. There are different forms of magnesium, but I recommend glycinate, citrate, threonate, or malate for headaches or migraines.

Curcumin 500–2000mg and Omega 3 Fatty acids 1000–2000mg daily—Because of their anti-inflammatory properties, research shows that curcumin and omega 3 fatty acids can decrease the severity and frequency of migraines.

Curcumin is best absorbed with Piperine (aka BioPerine), an extract from black pepper fruit added to supplements or healthy fats. You can even find it in liposomal form. It improves absorption through the fatty walls of your cell membranes.

EPA and DHA are the two types of Omega 3 fatty acids found in algae or fish sources. If you choose a fish oil supplement, make sure it is high quality because heavy metals, such as mercury, are found in fish. I recommend Nordic Naturals for fish or algae sources, because they are of excellent quality and ensure low levels of heavy metals. Vivo Life also has the cleanest algae Omega 3 that I have found. It has the least amount of ingredients and is in liquid form, if you don't mind the taste!

›› *Precautions: Avoid both supplements if you're on blood-thinning medications. Avoid curcumin if you are also on diabetic/blood sugar lowering medications, antacids, or certain antidepressants.*

Ginger—A study showed that ginger was just as effective as taking Sumatriptan (Imitrex) in treating migraines by decreasing the severity and pain. Another study showed a better response than the placebo in a double-blind study.

Ginger has anti-inflammatory properties, so it makes sense that it helps reduce pain and severity. You can find ginger in capsule form, tinctures, and teas. You can also make your own ginger tea by boiling the fresh ginger root in water.

›› *Precautions: Large doses of ginger may cause abdominal discomfort, heartburn, nausea, and diarrhea. Also, discuss taking ginger with your licensed medical provider if you are on any blood-thinning, diabetic, or high blood pressure medications.*

Essential oils—Lavender and peppermint essential oils mixed with a carrier oil such as coconut, almond, jojoba, can help relieve headaches. In addition, lavender has muscle relaxant and calming effects. Peppermint has anti-inflammatory benefits.

Apply diluted essential oils directly to your temples, forehead, and neck at the onset of a headache.

SUPPLEMENTS

Support Estrogen Metabolism

We're all different, and not all cases of estrogen dominance should be treated the same. Many resources and blogs on the internet recommend taking DIM (diindolylmethane) for estrogen dominance and hormonal imbalance. However, not everyone needs DIM. There are cases where DIM can actually make your symptoms worse. This is why it is vital to understand estrogen metabolism. Proper testing will uncover the phase of estrogen metabolism where you need support.

Here are the different phases with corresponding supplements to support each stage of estrogen metabolism.

PHASE I

DIM 200mg—DIM stands for diindolylmethane, a compound found in cruciferous vegetables such as broccoli, cauliflower, cabbage, bok choy, and kale. It helps support estrogen metabolism by increasing 2-OHE1. Studies show DIM can help reduce the risk of breast cancer which makes sense because it increases 2-OHE1.

›› *Precautions: Can cause headaches, worsening of menstrual cramps, nausea, vomiting, gas or diarrhea, if Phase I does not need support or the gut isn't healed.*

I3C 200mg—Indole-3-carbinole (I3C) is another compound found in cruciferous vegetables that also helps support the production of more 2-OHE1. You can take it separately or with DIM. Studies also show that I3C can help reduce the risk of breast cancer by increasing 2-OHE1.

›› *Precautions: I3C may increase bleeding, so it should be avoided if you have a bleeding disorder or are on blood-thinning medications.*

PHASE II

Broccoli sprout extract—Broccoli sprout extract contains sulforaphane which is a powerful antioxidant. It helps support estrogen metabolism in Phase II. It's also excellent to take in combination with DIM.

›› *Precautions: Broccoli sprout extract also does contain glucosinolates which can affect those with thyroid disorders.*

Folate 400–800mcg + Vitamin B12 500mcg—Vitamins B12 and Folate are essential for the methylation pathway, which protects and repairs DNA. They are also needed to support Phase II of estrogen metabolism. Remember, Phase II is where estrogen gets converted into its inactive form.

Many people have a genetic mutation called MTHFR which reduces the conversion of folic acid to folate. Because of this mutation, it is crucial to take the active form of folate, which is 5-methyltetrahydrofolate (5-MTHF). In addition, you also need the active form of Vitamin B12, which is methylcobalamin.

However, some people can over methylate and usually feel worse when taking these forms of vitamins. This is why it is important to check homocysteine to see if you need extra support.

If homocysteine is high, this is typically a sign of low Folate and Vitamin B12, which requires supplementation. Research has also shown that those with MTHFR mutations (A1298C and/or C677T) have an increased risk of miscarriage. Supplementation with Folate and Vitamin B12 are linked to lower rates of miscarriages.

To see if you have a mutation of either of these genes, I recommend the StrateGene test.

➤➤ *Precautions: Avoid supplements with folic acid because this form does not get converted into folate if you have an MTHFR genetic mutation.*

TMG 500mg + Choline 500mg daily—Trimethylglycine (TMG) and choline are methylation co-factors that may also be needed for methylation support. Unfortunately, these cannot be checked through routine blood work.

Thankfully, specialty functional medicine lab testing companies can check these levels. For example, Genova Diagnostics can run a Methylation Panel. This panel also determines if you have any other genetic mutations, in addition to MTHFR, that require the supplementation of these two co-factors.

TMG's plant food sources are beets, broccoli, shellfish, spinach, quinoa, and marine algae. In addition, choline is found in high amounts in eggs and animal meat. Plant foods sources of choline include almonds, cauliflower, broccoli, shiitake mushrooms, quinoa, kidney beans, and soybeans.

➤➤ *Precautions: TMG can increase bad cholesterol (LDL) in those who already have high cholesterol and even those who do not. It can also increase LDL in people who are obese or have kidney failure. In addition, there are different forms of choline, so check with your medical provider before taking if you have a blood clotting disorder, kidney disease, cardiovascular disease, or are taking blood-thinning or diabetic medications.*

Magnesium 200–400mg—I call magnesium the miracle mineral. It's been used for years to lower blood pressure, correct arrhythmias, asthma, reduce anxiety, and relieve constipation and cramps.

In addition, it acts as a natural muscle relaxant and is in over 300 metabolic pathways. It also regulates blood sugar, calms your nervous system, improves sleep, strengthens bones, and is essential for estrogen metabolism via the COMT gene, which is Phase II.

There are many different types of magnesium that result in different effects on the body:

* **Magnesium Oxide**: the most common type, but it has poor absorption, making it excellent for constipation.
* **Magnesium Citrate**: the most used and least expensive, has calming effects, and is a mild laxative.
* **Magnesium Malate**: best for muscle aches and pains, and chronic fatigue.
* **Magnesium Taurate**: best for cardiovascular support to protect the heart from damage and improve blood pressure, with no laxative effects.
* **Magnesium Threonate**: the only form of magnesium that crosses the blood-brain barrier, best for improving cognitive function and memory and preventing migraines.
* **Magnesium Glycinate**: the most bioavailable of them all and best absorbed, has calming effects and can improve sleep, may have mild laxative effects if you take too much.

You can take different types of magnesium, depending on the outcome you want. However, one company called BioOptimizers contains a combination of seven different types of magnesium, so you can get the benefits of multiple forms in just two capsules.

Resveratrol 200mg—I love this powerful antioxidant found in red fruit such as grapes, cranberries, and pomegranate. Resveratrol lowers 4-OHE1 by converting it to 4-Methoxyestrone (4-MeE1), which is not carcinogenic like 4-OHE1. Therefore it helps to reduce the risk of breast cancer.

I know what you're thinking, red wine can reduce the risk! It's possible because it does contain resveratrol. However, remember that alcohol depletes glutathione and negatively impacts estrogen metabolism. Therefore, it's better to eat the whole fruit and take in extra through a supplement. I recommend looking for a resveratrol supplement with an extract from Japanese knotweed.

›› *Precautions: Resveratrol could increase bleeding, so talk to your medical provider if you have a bleeding disorder, are on blood-thinning medication, or are about to have surgery. Even though it helps with estrogen metabolism, it may have weak estrogen effects, so it should be avoided in those with estrogen-positive breast, ovarian, and uterine cancer and used with caution in those with endometriosis and uterine fibroids.*

PHASE III

Calcium-d-glucarate 100–300mg—Calcium-d-glucarate (CDG) is produced in small amounts in our bodies but is also found in food such as apples, oranges, grapefruit, and cruciferous vegetables.

If the beta-glucuronidase enzyme gets produced in high amounts during Phase II because of imbalance in your gut, CDG does not actually lower beta-glucuronidase. Instead, CDG inhibits beta-glucuronidase from turning the inactive forms of estrogen back into their active form, so it does not get recirculated back into the body.

›› *Precautions: CDG may increase the breakdown of medications through your liver, such as Tylenol, Lipitor, Valium, Ativan, Lamictal, and Digoxin, which decreases the effectiveness of these medications. Alcohol also increases the metabolism of CDG and reduces its efficacy to inhibit beta-glucuronidase.*

Support Progesterone Production

For those with two estrogen dominant patterns with low progesterone, ED-2 and ED-3, natural supplements can help support progesterone production without taking progesterone replacement.

In fact, if women are still cycling, I prefer to support progesterone naturally and work on lifestyle factors before resorting to hormone replacement therapy. The exception is when it is proven that there is a genetic condition or a disorder that inhibits the production of progesterone. In this case, replacement is the only option.

Vitamin B6 25–50mg daily—Pyridoxine is Vitamin B6. Like all other B vitamins, it is water-soluble and cannot be stored by your body. Research shows B6 helps increase progesterone levels and reduces estrogen levels by supporting methylation in Phase II. Studies also show a reduction in miscarriage from supplementation with B6.

>> *Precautions: If you exceed 100mg daily, you may develop involuntary muscle contractions, painful or discolored skin lesions, heartburn, nausea, pins and needles sensation in your extremities, decreased sensation to pain and temperature, and/or sensitivity to light.*

Vitamin C 1000–2000mg daily—Vitamin C also helps your body to produce progesterone. However, I previously mentioned that your body can only absorb 250–500mg of Vitamin C at a time. So you're probably thinking, how do I get up to 1000–2000mg daily?

I recommend taking smaller doses throughout the day, such as 500mg 2–4 times a day, or buy Vitamin C in liposomal form. There are pros and cons to the liposomal form.

Pros: Like Curcumin, fat molecules encapsulate Vitamin C to help it cross our fatty cell membranes for better absorption. Better absorption means less goes to waste.

Cons: Vitamin C is usually synthetic and derived from corn in the form of ascorbic acid. Therefore, I recommend finding Vitamin C derived from citrus fruit, acerola cherry, camu camu, or rose hips. These also contain bioflavonoids such as rutin and hesperidin, which actually enhance the effects of Vitamin C.

>> *Precautions: Avoid if you have hemochromatosis because this increases the absorption of iron. High doses of Vitamin C in those with Glucose-6-phosphate dehydrogenase (G6PD) deficiency can cause hemolytic anemia.*

Vitex 500–1000mg daily—Vitex agnus-castus L. (aka Chaste Tree or Chasteberry) is a flowering herb that increases progesterone and relieves PMS symptoms. Vitex can also lower prolactin levels if elevated. However, an MRI of the brain for a pituitary tumor with elevated prolactin levels should be ruled out first.

>> *Precautions: Do not take Vitex if you have PCOS with high levels of LH. For example, if the FSH:LH ratio is 1:3 (should be 1:1). This can increase luteinizing hormone (LH), which could worsen PCOS. It may also have mild estrogenic effects, so do not take it if you have had estrogen or progesterone positive breast, uterine or endometrial cancer.*

Evening Primrose Oil 500–1000mg—Evening Primrose is a flowering herb. The oil extracted from its seeds increases progesterone levels. It also contains two omega 6 fatty acids, linoleic acid and gamma-linoleic acid. These both have anti-inflammatory effects and can help relieve PMS symptoms. However, most forms of evening primrose oil in capsule form are not vegan friendly, so you could take it in oil form and add it to a smoothie or shake.

>> *Precautions: Do not take if you have a bleeding or seizure disorder, and advise your provider if you are scheduled for surgery as this can increase bleeding.*

Bladderwrack—According to research, an edible brown seaweed called bladderwrack helps reduce estrogen and increase progesterone levels. In fact, Japanese women tend to have lower circulating estrogen levels primarily due to their diet, which is high in soy and seaweed. So be sure to have your thyroid levels monitored closely when taking this supplement.

>> *Precautions: Those with thyroid disorders, including hypothyroidism, Hashimoto's, hyperthyroidism, Grave's disease, and thyroid cancer, should avoid taking bladderwrack because it contains iodine.*

Adrenal Support
In addition to adding adaptation activities to your daily routine (see chapter 16), some supplements help support your adrenals by balancing out your cortisol levels.

In James Allen's book "*As A Man Thinketh*," he writes, "A change of diet will not help a man (or woman) who will not change his (or her) thoughts."

This applies to supplements too! You cannot expect to lower your cortisol levels with supplements alone. It is crucial to incorporate the adaptation activities and work on your mindset. Start by reframing and shifting your perspective about situations in your life.

Then while you work on your mindset, use supplements to help your adrenals adapt at a cellular level. Here are my recommended supplements for adrenal support.

Adaptogens

Adaptogens are herbs and mushrooms that help your body handle stress in a healthier way.

Herbs

Ashwagandha 300–600mg daily—This herb increases resilience to stress and reduces anxiety.
›› *Precautions: Do not take if you have autoimmune disorders such as Rheumatoid Arthritis and Lupus because it is in the nightshade family. Also, avoid it if you have a gastric ulcer or are taking blood pressure medications.*

Rhodiola 100–200mg daily—The root of this flowering herb helps improve mental focus and clarity. This may be a better, more natural form of Adderall for those with ADD/ADHD.
›› *Precautions: Rhodiola might increase the side effects of escitalopram when taken together. It can also affect the metabolism of some cholesterol, antifungal, and allergy medications.*

Eleuthero 200–400mg daily—Also known as Siberian ginseng. It can help provide cognitive support and increase energy if you have fatigue from stress.

›› *Precautions: Can cause a pounding or irregular heartbeat and high blood pressure. It may also have mild estrogenic effects, so do not take it if you have had estrogen or progesterone positive breast, uterine or endometrial cancer.*

Holy Basil 300–500mg daily—Also known as Tulsi, and is from the basil family. It helps reduce anxiety, depression and improve energy. It also has anti-aging properties because it is rich in antioxidants.

›› *Precautions: Holy basil can lower blood glucose, so diabetics should use this with caution and monitor their glucose levels. It can also lower thyroxine levels and worsen those with hypothyroidism.*

Bacopa 300mg daily—This herb also helps to reduce anxiety, depression, improve your memory, and lower cortisol levels.

›› *Precautions: It can slow down heart rate, so do not take it if your heart rate is already low (aka bradycardia). Bacopa can increase secretions which can worsen stomach ulcers, cause urinary obstruction, or lung conditions such as asthma or COPD. It should also be avoided with thyroid disorders and those on thyroid medication because it can increase thyroid hormone.*

Mushrooms

Many different adaptogenic mushrooms have their own unique benefits in helping your body adapt during stress.

Cordyceps—One of my favorite adaptogenic mushrooms that is known for its ability to increase energy, improve stamina, and support a healthy immune system.

Reishi—This mushroom also helps support your immune system and can help fight cancer because of it's anticancer and antioxidant properties. It helps your liver to neutralize toxins, relieves stress and anxiety, and can improve sleep.

Lion's Mane—When paired with rhodiola, this mushroom enhances brain function to improve mental focus and clarity. It also improves anxiety and depression, regenerates damaged nerve cells, fights cancer, improves cardiovascular health, and reduces inflammation.

Chaga—A nutrient-dense mushroom that contains vitamin D, iron, magnesium, potassium, manganese, and calcium. It helps relieve symptoms of stress and lower inflammation, blood sugar, and blood pressure.

Turkey tail—A colorful mushroom that actually looks like a turkey's tail. It helps support your immune and gut health by providing a great source of fiber to optimize healthy gut bacteria. It also improves the removal of toxins through the liver.

B Complex —I've already covered how B vitamins such as Folate, B12, and B6 support methylation and progesterone production. In addition, B vitamins are great for adrenal support by helping to reduce your cortisol response from stress. It also helps alleviate some symptoms, such as fatigue.

Vitamin C 1000–2000mg—Vitamin C is vital for adrenal support because your adrenal glands contain the highest amounts of Vitamin C. It is required for the production of neurotransmitters and steroid hormones that are produced by the adrenals. Those who have low cortisol levels are usually deficient in Vitamin C.

Liver Support
Here are also some great supplements and herbs that can help support detoxification and metabolism of estrogen and toxins in the liver.

N-Acetylcysteine (NAC) 600–900mg twice daily—NAC is the precursor to glutathione which helps protect your body from oxidative stress. It also fights against free radicals, supports detoxification of toxins through your liver, and protects your liver from damage from medications and toxins.

›› *Precautions: Could cause bronchospasm in people with asthma, increase bleeding and bruising in those with a bleeding disorder, and should be avoided before surgery. It can also cause drying of the mucus membranes, especially when taken long-term. Because of this, it should be avoided in those with Sjogren's Syndrome.*

Quercetin 100mg twice daily—This is a powerful antioxidant found in red onions, apples, and cherries. As I mentioned in Chapter 9, it has antihistamine effects and helps reduce liver inflammation and damage from free radicals.

›› *Precaution: Take caution if you have a sulfur allergy, as it contains a sulfur amino acid. It can also make kidney function worse in those with kidney disorders.*

Milk Thistle 300mg three times daily—This herb can help regenerate damaged liver cells and reduce damage to your liver caused by toxins.

›› *Precaution: Can trigger an allergic reaction to those allergic to the Asteraceae/Compositae plant family, including marigolds, daisies, chrysanthemums, and ragweed. It may also have mild estrogenic effects, so do not take it if you have had estrogen or progesterone positive breast, uterine or endometrial cancer.*

Dandelion root tea

The root from this herb has been found to have antioxidants that protect your liver and reduce inflammation. I recommend drinking 1–3 cups daily.

›› *Precaution: Can trigger an allergic reaction to those allergic to the Asteraceae/Compositae plant family including marigolds, daisies, chrysanthemums, and ragweed and/or have eczema. Also avoid it if you have a bleeding disorder, kidney failure, or are about to have surgery.*

Part IV

REBALANCING
YOUR ESTROGEN

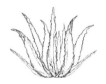

Chapter 20

MY BREAKTHROUGH 5-STEP PLAN

Congratulations! You made it to the last and most crucial section of this book. Hopefully, you have learned so much to this point.

Now is the time to put everything together! I created this 5-step plan to implement over 28 days, to break the cycle of menstrual agony so you can feel energized, sexy, and confident again.

In this plan, you'll find:
* Proper nutrients to support the production and metabolization of your hormones
* Tools for detoxifying your liver
* Information on seed cycling
* Exercises for your cycle
* Tips for creating a self-care practice

Even though you may not have a 28-day cycle, you can still use this as guidance for your own cycle. Just shorten or lengthen the number of days for each phase of your cycle to align with your own body's natural hormonal rhythms.

It doesn't matter if you have regular cycles, irregular cycles, take birth control, or have no cycles due to hypothalamic amenorrhea. You can still follow this plan!

If you have hypothalamic amenorrhea, continue to work with a licensed medical provider to determine the root cause, but ask them first if this plan is ok for you.

If you are on birth control, know that this plan will help you optimize your health. Though, you won't be able to fully rebalance your progesterone and estrogen until you stop taking it.

Preparing your body before coming off birth control can help your hormones return to balance. In addition, it will help lessen the side effects that come with suppressing your hormones long-term.

Now let's get into the 5 steps to start your journey to rebalancing your hormones.

STEP 1: TRACKING & SYNCHING YOUR CYCLE

It's essential to track your cycle. You need to know how long your total cycle is, how long your period lasts, and track changes in your cycles and symptoms over time. If you're not already tracking your cycle, I recommend downloading a cycle tracking app. See the resources section for recommendations.

If you aren't already, I also highly recommend syncing up with the moon and start with the New Moon or Full Moon.

If you're not sure which phase of the moon to sync with, tune into your energy. Is your energy at its lowest during the new moon or full moon?

Start with the phase where you feel your energy is at its lowest. To find out when is the next full or new moon, just ask Google or download a moon cycle app such as The Moon.

Seed Cycling

Perhaps you've never heard of seed cycling. Seed cycling can help women with irregular cycles sync back up with the moon. It can also help support a more regular cycle.

If you have regular cycles but severe PMS symptoms, seed cycling can help you feel better! The seeds themselves contain nutrients that help support the production and metabolization of estrogen and progesterone during each phase of your cycle.

For example, flax and pumpkin help support the production and metabolization of estrogen, which is vital in the first half of your menstrual cycle, the follicular phase.

Sesame and sunflower seeds help support progesterone production in the second half of the menstrual cycle, the luteal phase.

So how do you seed cycle? It's actually pretty simple. You can start the first day you start your period, or start with the next new moon if your cycle does not occur every month.

To begin seed cycling, purchase whole flax and pumpkin seeds and grind up 1 tablespoon fresh daily. Then, you can add the ground-up seeds to a shake, oatmeal, on top of sweet potatoes or salad.

Once one of my clients even got creative and mixed it in with her ground turkey.

Consume both types of seeds every day for 14 days, days 1–14 of a regular cycle.

Then on day 15, which should be around the full moon, you'll switch over and grind 1 tablespoon each of sesame and sunflower seeds.

Consume both of these seeds daily for another 14 days, days 15–28 of a regular cycle. Once you complete day 28 of the seed cycle, repeat it, even if you haven't started your period yet.

You will alternate the seeds every two weeks and do this for at least 3–4 months because it takes that long for your body to respond and regulate your hormones.

However, suppose you are still having irregular periods or PMS symptoms after 3 months. In that case, it means your hormones need to be tested to discover the additional support required for balance and to reduce your debilitating symptoms.

SEED CYCLING

❋ Days 1–14: Grind 1 tablespoon each of whole flax and pumpkin seed daily.

❋ Days 15–28: Grind 1 tablespoon each of whole sesame and sunflower seed daily.

❋ Then repeat after day 28 to start the seed cycle again.

›› *Note: I recommend grinding the seeds daily because they're usually rancid if you buy the pre-ground seeds. In addition, they do not contain the crucial nutrients for hormonal balance.*

STEP 2: EATING FOR YOUR CYCLE

Once you start tracking and syncing your cycle, you'll be able to follow my 28-day meal plan that supports each phase of your menstrual cycle.

Each week, I selected meals that contain the nutrients vital for each menstrual phase. They also support the production and metabolization of estrogen and progesterone.

Week 1: Menstrual —Because you are bleeding, you'll need to consume foods rich in iron and minerals.

Focus on foods high in iron such as almonds, beets, tofu, and beans, and sea vegetables which are full of minerals. Incorporate seeds for seed cycling, which are flax and pumpkin seeds.

Week 2: Follicular —During this phase, it's important to support estrogen metabolism in the liver and elimination in the gut as levels increase.

Increase vegetables and leafy greens, especially cruciferous vegetables. Add fermented foods, and healthy fats such as salmon, sardines, and olive oil. Continue consuming flax and pumpkin seeds.

Week 3: Ovulation —Since your energy is at it's highest, healthy fats and protein can help sustain your energy levels. Estrogen will have peaked and is starting to decline. Estrogen metabolism and elimination still needs to be supported during this phase.

Consume more foods high in healthy fat, fiber and protein, and low in carbs. Continue eating cruciferous vegetables, leafy greens. Also switch the seeds to sesame and sunflower seeds.

Week 4: Luteal—The uterus requires a lot of energy to get prepared for pregnancy. Plus your metabolism actually increases during this phase. Therefore, it is vital to increase slow burning carbohydrates. The result usually is cravings for sugar and processed foods. Progesterone is also produced, so certain foods help provide the necessary nutrients.

Consume more complex carbohydrates such as sweet potatoes, quinoa, or brown rice to reduce sugar cravings. Add foods high in Vitamin C, such as red peppers, berries, citrus fruit, and omega 3 foods such as salmon, nuts, seeds, and seaweed to support healthy progesterone levels. Eat foods high in magnesium such as dark chocolate, avocado, and pumpkin seeds. Continue sesame and sunflower seeds.

You can find the 28 day meal plan and recipes at:
www.estrogenisabtch.com/resources.

STEP 3: SELF CARE FOR YOUR CYCLE

We all need a little TLC, which is why it's essential to tune into your cycle to prioritize self-care.

If you've ever been on a plane, then you know the oxygen mask analogy: you have to put the mask on yourself before you can help anyone else. This excellent analogy not only applies to taking care of your health but also incorporating self-care into your daily routine.

So how can you show up fully for others if you're depleted and running on low reserves?

Menstrual Phase (3–7 days)—If you're tired, give yourself permission to take a nap, even if it's a 15–20 minute power nap. You can also book a massage or take an Epsom salt bath. Meditation is also very therapeutic during this time. It can help provide ideas and inspiration if you take some time to be still, even if it's for 5–10 minutes.

Late Follicular Phase (7–11 days)—This is a great time to get creative: color/paint, journal, learn something new, or start new projects. Also, spending time in nature can help boost your energy levels.

Ovulation (3–6 days)—Since your energy levels are at their highest, go out and have some fun! Hang out with your friends or go out on a date. This is also the best time to conceive if you are planning for pregnancy.

Luteal Phase (10–14 days)—As your energy levels start to decline, you may actually feel inspired to clear out some things in your life. Take this time to clean your home, take care of that to-do list, or get rid of clothes you haven't worn in over 5 years.

I recommend doing at least one of the self-care activities daily for each phase of the menstrual cycle. You must make time for these activities! They make a positive difference by helping your body adapt during stress and improving your day's outcome. I recommend setting a reminder on your phone or pencil it into your planner.

STEP 4: EXERCISING FOR YOUR CYCLE

Now that you've got down the tracking and meal planning and created a self-care practice, it's time to sync your exercise with your cycle. If you're a go-getter and want to start everything at once, by all means, go ahead! Steps 1–3 can be implemented simultaneously. However, if it is too much to do all at once, wait until your next cycle to start the exercises.

Menstrual Phase (3–7 days)—When you start your period, remember your energy levels will be at their lowest. Therefore, the best exercises during this time are low impact exercises such as walking, hiking, yoga, and pilates.

Late Follicular Phase (7–11 days)—Your energy levels increase once your period ends throughout the rest of your follicular phase. Start incorporating more moderate-intensity exercises like running, cycling, HIIT training, weight training, and body calisthenics.

Ovulation (3–6 days)—Your energy level is at its peak around ovulation. This is when you can exercise at a higher intensity like running, HIIT, and weight training. However, if you have any known adrenal dysfunction, it is best not to do high-intensity exercise. Instead, stick to low to moderate impact exercise even around ovulation.

Luteal Phase (10–14 days)—Once you move into the luteal phase, go back to low to moderate impact exercises such as jogging, swimming, walking, hiking, yoga, or pilates.

I recommend enjoying one of these exercises during each phase of your cycle for about 20 to 30 minutes, 3 to 4 times a week to start.

STEP 5: DETOX & REMOVE TOXINS

Detoxification

Since you learned that estrogens are metabolized in your liver first, then through your intestines, you might be thinking, "should I do a detox cleanse?"

Even though there are many juices, teas, and supplements for detoxing, the answer is no!

You see, your liver does a fantastic job at detoxing. So save your money and focus on these ways to support detoxification from your liver and through elimination from your intestines.

First, drink plenty of water each day. Your body removes toxins through sweat, urine, and poop. Water is vital for all of those mechanisms to occur; imagine that! Therefore, I recommend drinking at least half your body weight in ounces every day. So, for example, if you weigh 120 lbs, you'll want to drink at least 60 ounces or 7.5 cups of water daily.

Cruciferous vegetables are an excellent detox food. These include:
* Broccoli
* Cauliflower
* Cabbage
* Bok choy

Remember, these foods contain Indole-3-carbinol, which converts to DIM and sulforaphane. Remember that these compounds help support estrogen metabolism and detoxification from free radicals.

Free radicals are the by-products of waste that occur during metabolism or from chemical reactions in the body, which can cause damage to DNA and cancer.

Leafy greens are a great source of fiber that is important to help you stay regular.

Avocados and asparagus are excellent sources of glutathione, a powerful antioxidant produced by your liver. Glutathione is crucial to help support detoxification and rid your body of free radicals.

Citrus fruits contain antioxidants called flavonoids that upregulate your liver enzymes in Phase I and Phase II of estrogen detoxification. They also increase the good estrogen metabolite 2-hydroxyestrone.

Berries are another great source of fiber and polyphenols, both essential to support a healthy microbiome and keep you regular.

Soy helps reduce the harmful estrogen metabolite 4-hydroxyestrone production, which can be carcinogenic and promote breast cancer. Plus, soy contains antioxidants called isoflavones which also help reduce free radicals in the body.

Nuts and seeds, like leafy greens, are also a great source of fiber and help keep you regular. For example, flax seeds contain an insoluble fiber called lignin, which helps bind estrogen in your digestive tract. This enables your body to eliminate them in your bowel movements.

A sauna is another great way to support detoxification. Studies show that toxins and heavy metals exit your body through sweat. I recommend using a sauna at least 2–3 times a week for 10–15 minutes to start.

However, if you have breast implants and are scheduled for surgery, it is important to wait until after surgery, and you are cleared by your surgeon to use the sauna because you don't want toxins to be released before surgery.

Lastly, make sure you have regular bowel movements daily. Regularly getting rid of waste is important for Phase III of estrogen metabolism. Actually, it's vital for getting rid of toxins in general.

Check out the natural remedies to help support regular, daily bowel movements. If you are not going at least once a day and it's not the consistency of a soft log, not round pebbles, you need to check your gut.

Removing Toxins

The last thing to do as part of the 5 step plan is to remove the toxins you can control from your home.

Start by downloading the Think Dirty and Yuka app. Next, use the scanner to scan the barcode of personal care and other products in your home. This will give you an idea if there are any Half & Half or Dirty ingredients.

Since not all products have a barcode, you can also search by the product's name. If you don't find it in the apps, check Environmental Working Group's Skin Deep Database and search there.

Make a list of the products to keep and the products to replace. A bonus step is to research possible replacement products. For example, replace Lysol Power Bathroom Cleaner with Seventh Generation Tub & Tile Cleaner.

EWG also has a list of the Dozen Endocrine Disruptors in your home, such as plastic water bottles and food storage containers, and non-stick cookware. You can find this list at www.estrogenisabtch.com/resources.

Slowly start to swap these products for healthier alternatives. I included a few brands of cookware in the resources section at the end of this book.

You may find when you get to this step that swapping out a lot of products in your home may be overwhelming and costly, but don't sweat it! Just start with one or two things at a time.

Of course, I don't expect you to get rid of everything in your home in 28 days, as I definitely didn't. Yet at least you now have an awareness of what stays and what goes as you start transitioning to healthier products.

As I wrap up this section, I know it can seem overwhelming to implement everything at once, so I put 4 of these steps into a 28-day plan for you, including a meal plan and recipes.

This plan will help you see everything outlined week by week, synching your cycle, nutrition, self-care, and exercise. Remember, this is just a guide, and you have the choice whether you want to implement everything each week or one thing at a time and extend the plan out for 2–3 months.

I want to set you up for success, so know that it's ok to go at your own pace and do what feels right for you. You can find this plan at www.estrogenisabtch.com/resources.

Conclusion

Now that we have reached the end of this book, I hope you gained insight and knowledge about your hormones. You should also have a clear picture of what happens when estrogen becomes imbalanced. Finally, you now have simple steps to start implementing into your daily routine to take your health into your own hands.

Remember, the goal is not to completely get rid of estrogens. We need estrogen to help prepare the uterine lining, mature an egg for release, and protect your organs from chronic disorders.

However, you need to balance out the ratio of estrogen to progesterone, so estrogen isn't dominating anymore!

It's like the lessons we've learned from Goldilocks: we don't want too much or too little estrogen. Instead, we need a nice balance to function optimally without limitations and not miss out on life's most memorable moments anymore.

If we don't have the chance to work together, I highly recommend finding a functional medicine practitioner or naturopath in your area to guide you on your journey towards creating lasting change.

I want to acknowledge you for reading this book. You are showing up for yourself by learning. You're looking for other ways outside of conventional medicine to treat hormonal imbalances. We need more women like you to take a stand and be an advocate for their health!

I believe that once you take your health into your hands and rebalance your hormones, it creates a ripple effect in every area of your life. This includes your family, your career or business, relationships, finances, and more.

Know that I hear you and see you, as I too once struggled with the imbalances of my hormones. I want you to know that it is possible to naturally support your hormones.

You don't have to be a victim of your cycle every month.

When you follow these 5 steps, you'll gain more energy than you could have imagined. You'll have clear skin, a better mood, happy periods, enhanced libido, and feel confident in your body!

Let this book be your guide and leave you empowered, knowing that you can support your hormones to work with you...not against you. Together we can shift the perspective that estrogen is a b*tch to estrogen is your best friend!

Live with Intention and Be Radiant!

RESOURCES

TESTING

Lab Ranges for Serum Levels
Progesterone 15–25
Estrogen—no optimal range
P/E2 ratio 150–200
Total Testosterone 30–50
Free Testosterone 3–8
DHEA 200–380
TSH 1–2.5
Free T4 1.0–1.5
Free T3 3–4
TPO < 4
Thyroglobulin Antibodies < 1
Vitamin D 60–80
Magnesium RBC 5.5–6.5
Fasting Glucose: 70–85
Fasting Insulin: < 8

Adrenals & Hormones
DUTCH
Physician's Labs

Microbiome
Viome
Genova GI Effects
Doctor's Data GI MAP

HELPFUL APPS

Cycle Tracking
My Flo
Glow
Clue
Daysy

Meditation
Calm
Insight Timer
Headspace

Deep Breathing
Breethe
Breathwrk

Removing Toxins
Think Dirty app
Yuka app
EWG Skin Deep Database

BETTER PRODUCTS FOR YOUR BODY AND HOME

Kitchen cookware
Le Creuset
Carraway
GreenLife
Cast Iron
Stainless Steel

Cleaning Products
Household cleaner—Branch Basics, Blueland
Sponges—Blueland
Laundry Detergent—Rockin' Green

DIY All Purpose Cleaner
1 glass spray bottle from Grove
½ filtered water
½ distilled vinegar
10–20 drops of essential oils (I use lemon, tea tree, & peppermint)

Personal Care Product Brands
Soap—Dr. Bronner's
Shampoo—Native, 100% Pure, Annmarie Gianni
Moisturizer & Cleanser—Annmarie Gianni, 100% Pure
Makeup—100% Pure
Deodorant—Native

Period Products
Menstrual cups—made from medical-grade silicone, brands: Cora Cup,
Flex, Saalt, Organi Cup, Nixit
Tampons—Lola, Rael, L., Cora
Pads—Lola, Rael, L., Cora
Panties—Thinx, Knix

BOOKS

Stress Less, Accomplish More by Emily Fletcher
Beyond the Pill by Dr. Jolene Brighten
The 4 Phase Histamine Reset by Dr. Becky Campbell
The Hormone Reset by Dr. Sarah Gotfried
Dirty Genes by Dr. Ben Lynch
The Pantry Principle by Mira Dessy, NE

INFORMATIONAL

Breast Implant Illness
www.breastimplantilness.com
https://www.breastimplantsafetyalliance.org
https://www.breastimplanthealthsummit.com

FINDING A PRACTITIONER

Institute for Functional Medicine (IFM)—
www.ifm.org/find-a-practitioner

American Academy of Anti-Aging Medicine (A4M)—
www.a4m.com/find-a-doctor.html

American Association of Naturopath Physicians—
www.naturopathic.org/AF_MemberDirectory.asp?version=2

SCAN THE CODE

Online resources page for the 28 day plan, recipes, and more!

ACKNOWLEDGEMENTS

First I want to give God gratitude and praise because He has been guiding me every step of the way of my life and journey here on this Earth. This book and my work would not have been possible without God.

To my husband Joshua Vazquez who is my soulmate and my rock since we met in 2011. He believed in me before I even believed in myself and has been my number one cheerleader since starting Radiant Health. I am so grateful and appreciative of his never ending support to go above and beyond for us, so I can focus on the practice and writing this book.

To my parents, sisters, and my in-laws who have supported me when I started Radiant Health and are always providing feedback to help me grow and as I create exciting things to help empower and inspire women all over the world.

To my administrative assistant, Tamara Wilkinson-Chin, who has been a blessing from God to help me take care of the administrative tasks of the business so I can focus more time on creating and writing this book.

To Vanessa Lindo who is the amazing and talented designer who designed the book cover and the website for Radiant Health.

To Patti Lemene with her expertise and knowledge of layout and formatting, designed the beautiful interior of this book and brought it to life.

To Dr. Meghan Walker for the opportunity to be a part of her Mastermind, The Clinician Code, for clinician entrepreneurs. This book would not have been possible without being a part of this amazing group who have supported, encouraged, and provided me guidance every step of the way.

Lastly, I also want to give a special thanks to Katie Thomson Aitken and Kirstie Griffiths in The Clinician Code who have also written and self-published their own books, and their willingness and generosity to answer my questions about getting my first book self-published.

REFERENCES

What is ED?
Patel S, Homaei A, Raju AB, Meher BR. Estrogen: The necessary evil for human health, and ways to tame it. Biomed Pharmacother. 2018 Jun;102:403–411. doi: 10.1016/j.biopha.2018.03.078. Epub 2018 Mar 22. PMID: 29573619. PMID: 29573619

Symptoms of ED
Vorherr H. Fibrocystic breast disease: pathophysiology, pathomorphology, clinical picture, and management. Am J Obstet Gynecol. 1986 Jan;154(1):161–79. doi: 10.1016/0002-9378(86)90421-7. PMID: 3511705

Cavalieri E, Chakravarti D, Guttenplan J, Hart E, Ingle J, Jankowiak R, Muti P, Rogan E, Russo J, Santen R, Sutter T. Catechol estrogen quinones as initiators of breast and other human cancers: implications for biomarkers of susceptibility and cancer prevention. Biochim Biophys Acta. 2006 Aug;1766(1):63–78. Epub 2006 Apr 19. PMID: 16675129

Juhl CR, Bergholdt HKM, Miller IM, Jemec GBE, Kanters JK, Ellervik C. Dairy Intake and Acne Vulgaris: A Systematic Review and Meta-Analysis of 78,529 Children, Adolescents, and Young Adults. Nutrients. 2018;10(8):1049. Published 2018 Aug 9. PMID: 30096883

Causes of ED
Jane Houlihan, Timothy Kropp, Ph.D., Richard Wiles, Sean Gray, Chris Campbell. Body Burden: The Pollution in Newborns. Environmental Working Group. Published July 14, 2005. Accessed July 1st, 2021. https://www.ewg.org/research/body-burden-pollution-newborns

Personal Care Products Safety Act Would Improve Cosmetics Safety. Environmental Working Group. Accessed July 1st, 2021. https://www.ewg.org/personal-care-products-safety-act-would-improve-cosmetics-safety

LiverTox: Clinical and Research Information on Drug-Induced Liver Injury [Internet]. Bethesda (MD): National Institute of Diabetes and Digestive and Kidney Diseases; 2012-. Estrogens and Oral Contraceptives. [Updated 2020 May 28]

Kucharska A, Szmurło A, Sińska B. Significance of diet in treated and untreated acne vulgaris. Postepy Dermatol Alergol. 2016;33(2):81–86. PMID: 27279815

Types of Estrogen
Reyes MR, Sifuentes-Alvarez S, Lazalde B. Estrogens are potentially the only steroids with an antioxidant role in pregnancy: in vitro evidence. Acta Obstetricia et Gynecologica. 2006;85:1090-1093

Patel S, Homaei A, Raju AB, Meher BR. Estrogen: The necessary evil for human health, and ways to tame it. Biomed Pharmacother. 2018 Jun;102:403–411. doi: 10.1016/j.biopha.2018.03.078. Epub 2018 Mar 22. PMID: 29573619

Tulchinsky D, Frigoletto FD Jr, Ryan KJ, Fishman J. Plasma estetrol as an index of fetal well-being. J Clin Endocrinol Metab. 1975 Apr;40(4):560–7. doi: 10.1210/jcem-40-4-560. PMID: 805156

Cui J, Shen Y, Li R. Estrogen synthesis and signaling pathways during aging: from periphery to brain. Trends Mol Med. 2013;19(3):197–209. doi:10.1016/j.molmed.2012.12.007. PMID: 23348042

Estrogen Metabolism
Phang-Lyn S, Llerena VA. Biochemistry, Biotransformation. [Updated 2020 Sep 2]. In: StatPearls [Internet]. Treasure Island (FL): StatPearls Publishing; 2021 Jan-

Taioli, E., Im, A., Xu, X. et al. Comparison of estrogens and estrogen metabolites in human breast tissue and urine. Reprod Biol Endocrinol 8, 93 (2010). https://doi.org/10.1186/1477-7827-8-93

Tsuchiya Y, Nakajima M, Yokoi T. Cytochrome P450-mediated metabolism of estrogens and its regulation in human. Cancer Lett. 2005 Sep 28;227(2):115–24. doi: 10.1016/j.canlet.2004.10.007. Epub 2004 Nov 19. PMID: 16112414

Allocati, N., Masulli, M., Di Ilio, C. et al. Glutathione transferases: substrates, inhibitors and pro-drugs in cancer and neurodegenerative diseases.Oncogenesis 7, 8 (2018). https://doi.org/10.1038/s41389-017-0025-3

Cavalieri E, Chakravarti D, Guttenplan J, Hart E, Ingle J, Jankowiak R, Muti P, Rogan E, Russo J, Santen R, Sutter T. Catechol estrogen quinones as initiators of breast and other human cancers: implications for biomarkers of susceptibility and cancer prevention. Biochim Biophys Acta. 2006 Aug;1766(1):63-78. doi: 10.1016/j.bbcan.2006.03.001. Epub 2006 Apr 19. PMID: 16675129

Obi N, Vrieling A, Heinz J, Chang-Claude J. Estrogen metabolite ratio: Is the 2-hydroxyestrone to 16α-hydroxyestrone ratio predictive for breast cancer?. Int J Womens Health. 2011;3:37–51. Published 2011 Feb 8. doi:10.2147/IJWH.S7595. PMID: 21339936

Kwa M, Plottel CS, Blaser MJ, Adams S. The Intestinal Microbiome and Estrogen Receptor-Positive Female Breast Cancer. J Natl Cancer Inst. 2016;108(8):djw029. Published 2016 Apr 22. doi:10.1093/jnci/djw029

Reddy BS, Hanson D, Mangat S, Mathews L, Sbaschnig M, Sharma C, Simi B. Effect of high-fat, high-beef diet and of mode of cooking of beef in the diet on fecal bacterial enzymes and fecal bile acids and neutral sterols. J Nutr. 1980 Sep;110(9):1880-7. doi: 10.1093/jn/110.9.1880. PMID: 7411244

Domellof L, Darby L, Hanson D, Mathews L, Simi B, Reddy BS. Fecal sterols and bacterial beta-glucuronidase activity: a preliminary metabolic epidemiology study of healthy volunteers from Umea, Sweden, and metropolitan New York. Nutr Cancer. 1982;4(2):120–7. doi: 10.1080/01635588209513747. PMID: 6298751

Im A, Vogel VG, Ahrendt G, et al. Urinary estrogen metabolites in women at high risk for breast cancer. Carcinogenesis. 2009;30(9):1532–1535. doi:10.1093/carcin/bgp139. PMID: 19502596

Birth Control

Speroff L. The formulation of oral contraceptives: does the amount of estrogen make any clinical difference? Johns Hopkins Med J. 1982 May;150(5):170–6. PMID: 7043035

Wang Q, Würtz P, Auro K, et al. Effects of hormonal contraception on systemic metabolism: cross-sectional and longitudinal evidence. Int J Epidemiol. 2016;45(5):1445–1457. doi:10.1093/ije/dyw147

Claudia Panzer, Sarah Wise, Gemma Fantini, Dongwoo Kang, Ricardo Munarriz, Andre Guay, Irwin Goldstein. Impact of oral contraceptives on sex hormone-binding globulin and androgen levels: a retrospective study in women with sexual dysfunction. J Sex Med. 2006 Jan;3(1):104–13. Doi: 10.1111/j.1743-6109.2005.00198.x

Qin Wang, Peter Würtz, Kirsi Auro, Laure Morin-Papunen, Antti J Kangas, Pasi Soininen, Mika Tiainen, Tuulia Tynkkynen, Anni Joensuu, Aki S Havulinna, Kristiina Aalto, Marko Salmi, Stefan Blankenberg, Tanja Zeller, Jorma Viikari, Mika Kähönen, Terho Lehtimäki, Veikko Salomaa, Sirpa Jalkanen, Marjo-Riitta Järvelin, Markus Perola, Olli T Raitakari, Debbie A Lawlor, Johannes Kettunen, Mika Ala-Korpela, Effects of hormonal contraception on systemic metabolism: cross-sectional and longitudinal evidence, International Journal of Epidemiology, Volume 45, Issue 5, October 2016, Pages 1445–1457, https://doi.org/10.1093/ije/dyw147

Kowalska K, Ściskalska M, Bizoń A, Śliwińska-Mossoń M, Milnerowicz H. Influence of oral contraceptives on lipid profile and paraoxonase and commonly hepatic enzymes activities. J Clin Lab Anal. 2018;32(1):e22194. doi:10.1002/jcla.22194

Khalili H. Risk of Inflammatory Bowel Disease with Oral Contraceptives and Menopausal Hormone Therapy: Current Evidence and Future Directions. Drug Saf. 2016 Mar;39(3):193–7. doi: 10.1007/s40264-015-0372-y. PMID: 26658991; PMCID: PMC4752384

Khalili H, Granath F, Smedby KE, et al. Association Between Long-term Oral Contraceptive Use and Risk of Crohn's Disease Complications in a Nationwide Study. Gastroenterology. 2016;150(7):1561–1567.e1. doi:10.1053/j.gastro.2016.02.041. PMID: 26919969

Vighi G, Marcucci F, Sensi L, Di Cara G, Frati F. Allergy and the gastro-intestinal system. Clin Exp Immunol. 2008;153 Suppl 1(Suppl 1):3–6. doi:10.1111/j.1365–2249.2008.03713.x

Bischoff SC, Barbara G, Buurman W, Ockhuizen T, Schulzke JD, Serino M, Tilg H, Watson A, Wells JM. Intestinal permeability—a new target for disease prevention and therapy. BMC Gastroenterol. 2014 Nov 18;14:189. doi: 10.1186/s12876-014-0189-7. PMID: 25407511; PMCID: PMC4253991

Fukui H. Increased Intestinal Permeability and Decreased Barrier Function: Does It Really Influence the Risk of Inflammation? Inflamm Intest Dis. 2016;1(3):135–145. doi:10.1159/000447252

Njeze GE. Gallstones. Niger J Surg. 2013;19(2):49–55. doi:10.4103/1117-6806.119236

Etminan M, Delaney JA, Bressler B, Brophy JM. Oral contraceptives and the risk of gallbladder disease: a comparative safety study. CMAJ. 2011;183(8):899–904. doi:10.1503/cmaj.110161

Atousa Aminzadeh, Ali Sabeti Sanat, and Saeed Nik Akhtar. Frequency of Candidiasis and Colonization of Candida albicans in Relation to Oral Contraceptive Pills. Iran Red Crescent Med J. 2016 Oct; 18(10): e38909. Published online 2016 Aug 17. doi: 10.5812/ircmj.38909. PMID: 28184328

Gut Health

Lichten E. Are the estrogenic hormonal effects of environmental toxins affecting small intestinal bacterial and microfilaria overgrowth? Med Hypotheses. 2017 Nov;109:90–94. doi: 10.1016/j.mehy.2017.09.022. Epub 2017 Sep 28. PMID: 29150304

Dukowicz AC, Lacy BE, Levine GM. Small intestinal bacterial overgrowth: a comprehensive review. Gastroenterol Hepatol (N Y). 2007;3(2):112–122. PMC3099351

Sachdev AH, Pimentel M. Gastrointestinal bacterial overgrowth: pathogenesis and clinical significance. Ther Adv Chronic Dis. 2013;4(5):223–231. doi:10.1177/2040622313496126

Wang SX, Wu WC. Effects of psychological stress on small intestinal motility and bacteria and mucosa in mice. World J Gastroenterol. 2005;11(13):2016–2021. doi:10.3748/wjg.v11.i13.2016. PMC4305729

Theisen, J., Nehra, D., Citron, D. et al. Suppression of gastric acid secretion in patients with gastroesophageal reflux disease results in gastric bacterial overgrowth and deconjugation of bile acids. J Gastrointest Surg 4, 50–54 (2000). https://doi.org/10.1016/S1091-255X(00)80032-3

Sarker SA, Ahmed T, Brüssow H. Hunger and microbiology: is a low gastric acid-induced bacterial overgrowth in the small intestine a contributor to malnutrition in developing countries?. Microb Biotechnol. 2017;10(5):1025–1030. doi:10.1111/1751-7915.12780

Patil AD. Link between hypothyroidism and small intestinal bacterial overgrowth. Indian J Endocrinol Metab. 2014;18(3):307–309. doi:10.4103/2230-8210.131155

Ernesto Cristiano Lauritano, Anna Lisa Bilotta, Maurizio Gabrielli, Emidio Scarpellini, Andrea Lupascu, Antonio Laginestra, Marialuisa Novi, Sandra Sottili, Michele Serricchio, Giovanni Cammarota, Giovanni Gasbarrini, Alfredo Pontecorvi, Antonio Gasbarrini, Association between Hypothyroidism and Small Intestinal Bacterial Overgrowth, The Journal of Clinical Endocrinology & Metabolism, Volume 92, Issue 11, 1 November 2007, Pages 4180–4184, https://doi.org/10.1210/jc.2007-0606

Reddymasu SC, McCallum RW. Small intestinal bacterial overgrowth in gastroparesis: are there any predictors? J Clin Gastroenterol. 2010 Jan;44(1):e8-13. doi: 10.1097/MCG.0b013e3181aec746. PMID: 20027008

Yan LH, Mu B, Pan D, et al. Association between small intestinal bacterial overgrowth and beta-cell function of type 2 diabetes. J Int Med Res. 2020;48(7):300060520937866. PMID: 32691685

Rana SV, Malik A, Bhadada SK, Sachdeva N, Morya RK, Sharma G. Malabsorption, Orocecal Transit Time and Small Intestinal Bacterial Overgrowth in Type 2 Diabetic Patients: A Connection. Indian J Clin Biochem. 2017 Mar;32(1):84–89. doi: 10.1007/s12291-016-0569-6. Epub 2016 May 3. PMID: 28149017

Petrone P, Sarkisyan G, Coloma E, Akopian G, Ortega A, Kaufman HS. Small Intestinal Bacterial Overgrowth in Patients With Lower Gastrointestinal Symptoms and a History of Previous Abdominal Surgery. Arch Surg.2011;146(4):444–447. doi:10.1001/archsurg.2011.55

Hua Chu, Mark Fox, Xia Zheng, Yanyong Deng, Yanqin Long, Zhihui Huang, Lijun Du, Fei Xu, Ning Dai, "Small Intestinal Bacterial Overgrowth in Patients with Irritable Bowel Syndrome: Clinical Characteristics, Psychological Factors, and Peripheral Cytokines",Gastroenterology Research and Practice, vol. 2016, Article ID 3230859, 8 pages,2016. https://doi.org/10.1155/2016/3230859

Kwa M, Plottel CS, Blaser MJ, Adams S. The Intestinal Microbiome and Estrogen Receptor-Positive Female Breast Cancer. J Natl Cancer Inst. 2016;108(8):djw029. Published 2016 Apr 22. doi:10.1093/jnci/djw029

Njeze GE. Gallstones. Niger J Surg. 2013;19(2):49–55. doi:10.4103/1117-6806.119236

Liu X, Xue R, Yang C, Gu J, Chen S, Zhang S. Cholestasis-induced bile acid elevates estrogen level via farnesoid X receptor-mediated suppression of the estrogen sulfotransferase SULT1E1. J Biol Chem. 2018;293(33):12759-12769. doi:10.1074/jbc.RA118.001789. PMC6102144

Wang HH, Liu M, Clegg DJ, Portincasa P, Wang DQ. New insights into the molecular mechanisms underlying effects of estrogen on cholesterol gallstone formation. Biochim Biophys Acta. 2009;1791(11):1037–1047. doi:10.1016/j.bbalip.2009.06.006. PMC2756670

Aminzadeh A, Sabeti Sanat A, Nik Akhtar S. Frequency of Candidiasis and Colonization of Candida albicans in Relation to Oral Contraceptive Pills. Iran Red Crescent Med J. 2016;18(10):e38909. Published 2016 Aug 17. doi:10.5812/ircmj.38909. PMC5291939

Spinillo A, Capuzzo E, Nicola S, Baltaro F, Ferrari A, Monaco A. The impact of oral contraception on vulvovaginal candidiasis. Contraception. 1995 May;51(5):293–7. doi: 10.1016/0010-7824(95)00079-p. PMID: 7628203

Lin XL, Li Z, Zuo XL. [Study on the relationship between vaginal and intestinal candida in patients with vulvovaginal candidiasis]. Zhonghua Fu Chan Ke Za Zhi. 2011 Jul;46(7):496–500. Chinese. PMID: 22041440

Amabebe E, Anumba DOC. The Vaginal Microenvironment: The Physiologic Role of Lactobacilli. Front Med (Lausanne). 2018;5:181. Published 2018 Jun 13. doi:10.3389/fmed.2018.00181. PMC: 6008313

Cheng G, Yeater KM, Hoyer LL. Cellular and molecular biology of Candida albicans estrogen response. Eukaryot Cell. 2006;5(1):180–191. doi:10.1128/EC.5.1.180-191.2006. PMC1360257

Insulin Resistance

Freeman AM, Pennings N. Insulin Resistance. [Updated 2020 Jul 10]. In: StatPearls [Internet]. Treasure Island (FL): StatPearls Publishing; 2021 Jan-. PMID: 29939616

Gavin KM, Cooper EE, Raymer DK, Hickner RC. Estradiol effects on subcutaneous adipose tissue lipolysis in premenopausal women are adipose tissue depot specific and treatment dependent. Am J Physiol Endocrinol Metab. 2013 Jun 1;304(11):E1167–74. doi: 10.1152/ajpendo.00023.2013. Epub 2013 Mar 26. PMID: 23531620

Adam TC, Hasson RE, Ventura EE, et al. Cortisol is negatively associated with insulin sensitivity in overweight Latino youth. J Clin Endocrinol Metab. 2010;95(10):4729–4735. doi:10.1210/jc.2010-0322. PMID: 20660036

Geer EB, Islam J, Buettner C. Mechanisms of glucocorticoid-induced insulin resistance: focus on adipose tissue function and lipid metabolism. Endocrinol Metab Clin North Am. 2014;43(1):75–102. doi:10.1016/j.ecl.2013.10.005. PMID: 24582093

Glucogenic Amino Acids. In: Encyclopedia of Genetics, Genomics, Proteomics and Informatics. Springer, Dordrecht. (2008) https://doi.org/10.1007/978-1-4020-6754-9_6938

Stress and Adrenals

McCorry LK. Physiology of the autonomic nervous system. Am J Pharm Educ. 2007;71(4):78. PMID: 17786266

Nerurkar A, Bitton A, Davis RB, Phillips RS, Yeh G. When physicians counsel about stress: results of a national study. JAMA Intern Med. 2013;173(1):76–77. PMID: 23403892

Ranabir S, Reetu K. Stress and hormones. Indian J Endocrinol Metab. 2011;15(1):18–22. PMID: 21584161

Berg JM, Tymoczko JL, Stryer L. Important Derivatives of Cholesterol Include Bile Salts and Steroid Hormones. Biochemistry. 5th edition. New York: W H Freeman; 2002. Section 26.4

Thyroid

Peeters RP, Visser TJ. Metabolism of Thyroid Hormone. [Updated 2017 Jan 1]. In: Feingold KR, Anawalt B, Boyce A, et al., editors. Endotext [Internet]. South Dartmouth (MA): MDText.com, Inc.; 2000

Salvatore Benvenga, Giovanni Capodicasa, Sarah Perelli, Roberto Vita. Support for the upregulation of serum thyrotropin by estrogens coming from the increased requirement of levothyroxine in one gynecomastic patient with excess of thyroxine-binding globulin secondary to exposure to exogenous estrogens. Journal of Clinical and Translational Endocrinology: Case Reports. 2018;10:21-24. ISSN 2214-6245. https://doi.org/10.1016/j.jecr.2018.10.001

Ana Paula Santin, Tania Weber Furlanetto. Role of Estrogen in Thyroid Function and Growth Regulation. Journal of Thyroid Research. 2011;2011:875125. PMID: 21687614

Norman A. Mazer. Interaction of Estrogen Therapy and Thyroid Hormone Replacement in Postmenopausal Women. Thyroid. 2004; 14:27–34

Marine Peyneau, Niloufar Kavian, Sandrine Chouzenoux, Carole Nicco, Mohamed Jeljeli, Laurie Toullec, Jeanne Reboul-Marty, Camille Chenevier-Gobeaux, Fernando M. Reis, Pietro Santulli, Ludivine Doridot, CharlesChapron, Frédéric Batteux. Role of thyroid dysimmunity and thyroid hormones in endometriosis. Proceedings of the National Academy of Sciences. Jun 2019;116 (24):11894–11899; DOI:10.1073/pnas.1820469116

Monteiro R, Teixeira D, Calhau C. Estrogen signaling in metabolic inflammation. Mediators Inflamm. 2014;2014:615917. doi:10.1155/2014/615917

Arduc A, Aycicek Dogan B, Bilmez S, Imga Nasiroglu N, Tuna MM, Isik S, Berker D, Guler S. High prevalence of Hashimoto's thyroiditis in patients with polycystic ovary syndrome: does the imbalance between estradiol and progesterone play a role? Endocr Res. 2015;40(4):204–10. PMID: 25822940

Histamine Intolerance

Mori H, Matsuda K, Yamawaki M, Kawata M. Estrogenic regulation of histamine receptor subtype H1 expression in the ventromedial nucleus of the hypothalamus in female rats. PLoS One. 2014;9(5):e96232. Published 2014 May 7. doi:10.1371/journal.pone.0096232. PMID: 24805361

Comas-Basté O, Sánchez-Pérez S, Veciana-Nogués MT, Latorre-Moratalla M, Vidal-Carou MDC. Histamine Intolerance: The Current State of the Art. Biomolecules. 2020;10(8):1181. Published 2020 Aug 14. doi:10.3390/biom10081181. PMID: 32824107

Bonds RS, Midoro-Horiuti T. Estrogen effects in allergy and asthma. Curr Opin Allergy Clin Immunol. 2013;13(1):92–99. doi:10.1097/ACI.0b013e32835a6dd6. PMID: 23090385

Passani M. Beatrice, Panula Pertti, Lin Jian-Sheng. Histamine in the brain. Frontiers in Systems Neuroscience. 2014;8:64. doi:10.3389/fnsys.2014.00064

Estrogen Dominant Conditions

Marquardt RM, Kim TH, Shin JH, Jeong JW. Progesterone and Estrogen Signaling in the Endometrium: What Goes Wrong in Endometriosis? Int J Mol Sci. 2019 Aug 5;20(15):3822. doi: 10.3390/ijms20153822. PMID: 31387263

Garavaglia E, Audrey S, Annalisa I, et al. Adenomyosis and its impact on women fertility. Iran J Reprod Med. 2015;13(6):327–336

Michael Fanta. Is polycystic ovary syndrome, a state of relative estrogen excess, a real risk factor for estrogen-dependant malignancies?, Gynecological Endocrinology, 29:2, 145–147, DOI: 10.3109/09513590.2012.730575

Patel S, Homaei A, Raju AB, Meher BR. Estrogen: The necessary evil for human health, and ways to tame it. Biomed Pharmacother. 2018 Jun;102:403–411. doi: 10.1016/j.biopha.2018.03.078. Epub 2018 Mar 22. PMID: 29573619

Dumitrescu R, Mehedintu C, Briceag I, Purcarea VL, Hudita D. The polycystic ovary syndrome: an update on metabolic and hormonal mechanisms. J Med Life. 2015;8(2):142–145

Bartolone L, Smedile G, Arcoraci V, Trimarchi F, Benvenga S. Extremely high levels of estradiol and testosterone in a case of polycystic ovarian syndrome. Hormone and clinical similarities with the phenotype of the alpha estrogen receptor null mice. J Endocrinol Invest. 2000 Jul–Aug;23(7):467–72. doi: 10.1007/BF03343757. PMID: 11005272

Moeloek FA, Moegny E. Endometriosis and luteal phase defect. Asia Oceania J Obstet Gynaecol. 1993 Jun;19(2):171–6. doi: 10.1111/j.1447-0756.1993.tb00369.x. PMID: 8379865

Joseph-Horne R, Mason H, Batty S, White D, Hillier S, Urquhart M, Franks S. Luteal phase progesterone excretion in ovulatory women with polycystic ovaries. Hum Reprod. 2002 Jun;17(6):1459–63. doi: 10.1093/humrep/17.6.1459. PMID: 12042261

Infertility

Chantalat E, Valera MC, Vaysse C, et al. Estrogen Receptors and Endometriosis. Int J Mol Sci. 2020;21(8):2815. Published 2020 Apr 17. doi:10.3390/ijms21082815

Findlay JK, Liew SH, Simpson ER, Korach KS. Estrogen signaling in the regulation of female reproductive functions. Handb Exp Pharmacol. 2010;(198):29–35. PMID: 20839084

Ozkan S, Murk W, Arici A. Endometriosis and infertility: epidemiology and evidence-based treatments. Ann N Y Acad Sci. 2008 Apr;1127:92–100. doi: 10.1196/annals.1434.007. PMID: 18443335

Marquardt RM, Kim TH, Shin JH, Jeong JW. Progesterone and Estrogen Signaling in the Endometrium: What Goes Wrong in Endometriosis? Int J Mol Sci. 2019 Aug 5;20(15):3822. doi: 10.3390/ijms20153822. PMID: 31387263; PMCID: PMC6695957

Macer ML, Taylor HS. Endometriosis and infertility: a review of the pathogenesis and treatment of endometriosis-associated infertility. Obstet Gynecol Clin North Am. 2012;39(4):535–549. doi:10.1016/j. ogc.2012.10.002

Garavaglia E, Audrey S, Annalisa I, et al. Adenomyosis and its impact on women fertility. Iran J Reprod Med. 2015;13(6):327–336

Autoimmune

Angum F, Khan T, Kaler J, Siddiqui L, Hussain A. The Prevalence of Autoimmune Disorders in Women: A Narrative Review. Cureus. 2020;12(5):e8094. Published 2020 May 13. doi:10.7759/cureus.8094

Rainer H. Straub, The Complex Role of Estrogens in Inflammation, Endocrine Reviews, Volume 28, Issue 5, 1 August 2007, Pages 521–574, https://doi.org/10.1210/er.2007–0001

Tang ZR, Zhang R, Lian ZX, Deng SL, Yu K. Estrogen-Receptor Expression and Function in Female Reproductive Disease. Cells. 2019;8(10):1123. Published 2019 Sep 21. doi:10.3390/cells8101123

Khan Deena, Ansar Ahmed S. The Immune System Is a Natural Target for Estrogen Action: Opposing Effects of Estrogen in Two Prototypical Autoimmune Diseases. Frontiers in Immunology. 2016;6:635. DOI=10.3389/fimmu.2015.00635

Cutolo M, Capellino S, Sulli A, Serioli B, Secchi ME, Villaggio B, Straub RH. Estrogens and autoimmune diseases. Ann N Y Acad Sci. 2006 Nov;1089:538-47. doi: 10.1196/annals.1386.043. PMID: 17261796

Arduc A, Aycicek Dogan B, Bilmez S, Imga Nasiroglu N, Tuna MM, Isik S, Berker D, Guler S. High prevalence of Hashimoto's thyroiditis in patients with polycystic ovary syndrome: does the imbalance between estradiol and progesterone play a role? Endocr Res. 2015;40(4):204–10. PMID: 25822940

Castagnetta LA, Carruba G, Granata OM, Stefano R, Miele M, Schmidt M, Cutolo M, Straub RH. Increased estrogen formation and estrogen to androgen ratio in the synovial fluid of patients with rheumatoid arthritis. J Rheumatol. 2003 Dec;30(12):2597-605. PMID: 14719200

Cutolo M, Villaggio B, Seriolo B, Montagna P, Capellino S, Straub RH, Sulli A. Synovial fluid estrogens in rheumatoid arthritis. Autoimmun Rev. 2004 Mar;3(3):193-8. doi: 10.1016/j.autrev.2003.08.003. PMID: 15110231

J. Rovensky, R. Kvetnansky, Z. Radikova, R. Imrich, O. Greguska, M. Viga, L. Macho. Hormone concentrations in synovial fluid of patients with rheumatoid arthritis. Clinical and Experimental Rheumatology. 2005; 23: 292–296.Song YW, Kang EH. Autoantibodies in rheumatoid arthritis: rheumatoid factors and anticitrullinated protein antibodies. QJM. 2010;103(3):139–146. doi:10.1093/qjmed/hcp165. PMID: 19926660

Arvikar SL, Crowley JT, Sulka KB, Steere AC. Autoimmune Arthritides, Rheumatoid Arthritis, Psoriatic Arthritis, or Peripheral Spondyloarthritis Following Lyme Disease. Arthritis Rheumatol. 2017;69(1):194–202. doi:10.1002/art.39866. PMID: 27636905

Maidhof W, Hilas O. Lupus: an overview of the disease and management options. P T. 2012;37(4):240–249. PMID: 22593636

Berger A. Th1 and Th2 responses: what are they?. BMJ. 2000;321(7258):424. doi:10.1136/bmj.321.7258.424

Desai MK, Brinton RD. Autoimmune Disease in Women: Endocrine Transition and Risk Across the Lifespan. Front Endocrinol (Lausanne). 2019;10:265. Published 2019 Apr 29. PMID: 31110493

Hill, L., Jeganathan, V., Chinnasamy, P. et al. Differential Roles of Estrogen Receptors αand β in Control of B-Cell Maturation and Selection. Mol Med 17, 211–220 (2011)

Lourenço EV, La Cava A. Cytokines in systemic lupus erythematosus. Curr Mol Med. 2009;9(3):242–254. PMID: 19355907

Breast Implant Illness

Kaplan J, Rohrich R. Breast implant illness: a topic in review. Gland Surg. 2021;10(1):430–443. doi:10.21037/gs-20-231

Kappel, Rita & Boer, Lucas & Dijkman, Henry. Gel Bleed and Rupture of Silicone Breast Implants Investigated by Light-, Electron Microscopy and Energy Dispersive X-ray Analysis of Internal Organs and Nervous Tissue. Clin Med Rev. 2016, 3:087

Wee CE, Younis J, Isbester K, et al. Understanding Breast Implant Illness, Before and After Explantation: A Patient-Reported Outcomes Study. Ann Plast Surg. 2020;85(S1 Suppl 1):S82-S86. doi:10.1097/SAP.0000000000002446

Pollack AZ, Schisterman EF, Goldman LR, et al. Cadmium, lead, and mercury in relation to reproductive hormones and anovulation in pre-menopausal women. Environ Health Perspect. 2011;119(8):1156–1161. doi:10.1289/ehp.1003284. PMID: 21543284

Kevin M. Rice, Ernest M. Walker Jr, Miaozong Wu, Chris Gillette, Eric R. Blough. Environmental Mercury and Its Toxic Effects. Journal of Preventive Medicine and Public Health. 2014; 47(2): 74–83

Breast Cancer

BRCA Gene Mutations: Cancer Risk and Genetic Testing. National Cancer Institute. Reviewed November 19, 2020. Accessed July 10th, 2021. https://www.cancer.gov/about-cancer/causes-prevention/genetics/brca-fact-sheet

Kell MR, Burke JP. Management of breast cancer in women with BRCA gene mutation. BMJ. 2007;334(7591):437–438. doi:10.1136/bmj.39114.354248.80

Taioli, E., Im, A., Xu, X. et al. Comparison of estrogens and estrogen metabolites in human breast tissue and urine. Reprod Biol Endocrinol 8, 93 (2010). https://doi.org/10.1186/1477-7827-8-93

Cavalieri E, Chakravarti D, Guttenplan J, Hart E, Ingle J, Jankowiak R, Muti P, Rogan E, Russo J, Santen R, Sutter T. Catechol estrogen quinones as initiators of breast and other human cancers: implications for biomarkers of susceptibility and cancer prevention. Biochim Biophys Acta. 2006 Aug;1766(1):63–78. doi: 10.1016/j.bbcan.2006.03.001. Epub 2006 Apr 19. PMID: 16675129

Kwa M, Plottel CS, Blaser MJ, Adams S. The Intestinal Microbiome and Estrogen Receptor-Positive Female Breast Cancer. J Natl Cancer Inst. 2016;108(8):djw029. Published 2016 Apr 22. doi:10.1093/jnci/djw029. PMID: 27107051

Alan A. Arslan, Karen L. Koenig, Per Lenner, Yelena Afanasyeva, Roy E. Shore, Yu Chen, EvaLundin, Paolo Toniolo, Göran Hallmans and Anne Zeleniuch-Jacquotte. Circulating Estrogen Metabolites and Risk of Breast Cancer in Postmenopausal Women. Cancer Epidemiol Biomarkers. Prev July 1 2014 (23) (7) 1290–1297; DOI:10.1158/1055-9965.EPI-14-0009

Obi N, Vrieling A, Heinz J, Chang-Claude J. Estrogen metabolite ratio: Is the 2-hydroxyestrone to 16α-hydroxyestrone ratio predictive for breast cancer?. Int J Womens Health. 2011;3:37-51. Published 2011 Feb 8. doi:10.2147/IJWH.S7595

Jiang Y, Gong P, Madak-Erdogan Z, et al. Mechanisms enforcing the estrogen receptor β selectivity of botanical estrogens. FASEB J. 2013;27(11):4406–4418. doi:10.1096/fj.13-234617

Morito K, Hirose T, Kinjo J, Hirakawa T, Okawa M, Nohara T, Ogawa S, Inoue S, Muramatsu M, Masamune Y. Interaction of phytoestrogens with estrogen receptors alpha and beta. Biol Pharm Bull. 2001 Apr;24(4):351–6. doi: 10.1248/bpb.24.351. PMID: 11305594

Messina, M.J., Wood, C.E. Soy isoflavones, estrogen therapy, and breast cancer risk: analysis and commentary. Nutr J 7, 17 (2008). https://doi. org/10.1186/1475-2891-7-17

Santin AP, Furlanetto TW. Role of estrogen in thyroid function and growth regulation. J Thyroid Res. 2011;2011:875125. doi:10.4061/2011/875125. PMID: 21687614

Rodriguez AC, Blanchard Z, Maurer KA, Gertz J. Estrogen Signaling in Endometrial Cancer: a Key Oncogenic Pathway with Several Open Questions. Horm Cancer. 2019;10(2–3):51–63. doi:10.1007/s12672-019-0358-9. PMID: 30712080

Hsu LH, Chu NM, Kao SH. Estrogen, Estrogen Receptor and Lung Cancer. Int J Mol Sci. 2017;18(8):1713. Published 2017 Aug 5. doi:10.3390/ijms18081713. PMID: 28783064

Bado I, Gugala Z, Fuqua SAW, Zhang XH. Estrogen receptors in breast and bone: from virtue of remodeling to vileness of metastasis. Oncogene. 2017;36(32):4527–4537. doi:10.1038/onc.2017.94. PMID: 28368409

Caiazza F, Ryan EJ, Doherty G, Winter DC, Sheahan K. Estrogen receptors and their implications in colorectal carcinogenesis. Front Oncol. 2015;5:19. Published 2015 Feb 2. doi:10.3389/fonc.2015.00019. PMID: 25699240

Mungenast F, Thalhammer T. Estrogen biosynthesis and action in ovarian cancer. Front Endocrinol (Lausanne). 2014;5:192. Published 2014 Nov 12. doi:10.3389/fendo.2014.00192. PMID: 25429284

Godinho-Mota JCM, Gonçalves LV, Mota JF, et al. Sedentary Behavior and Alcohol Consumption Increase Breast Cancer Risk Regardless of Menopausal Status: A Case-Control Study. Nutrients. 2019;11(8):1871. Published 2019 Aug 12. doi:10.3390/nu11081871

Xenoestrogens

Paterni I, Granchi C, Minutolo F. Risks and benefits related to alimentary exposure to xenoestrogens. Crit Rev Food Sci Nutr. 2017;57(16):3384–3404. doi:10.1080/10408398.2015.1126547. PMID: 26744831

Fucic A, Gamulin M, Ferencic Z, et al. Environmental exposure to xenoestrogens and oestrogen related cancers: reproductive system, breast, lung, kidney, pancreas, and brain. Environ Health. 2012;11 Suppl 1(Suppl 1):S8. Published 2012 Jun 28. doi:10.1186/1476-069X-11-S1-S8. PMID: 22759508

Piergiorgio La Rosa, Marco Pellegrini, Pierangela Totta, Filippo Acconcia, Maria Marino. Xenoestrogens Alter Estrogen Receptor (ER) α Intracellular Levels. PLOS ONE. 2014;9(5): e99379.https://doi.org/10.1371/journal.pone.0099379

Chan Jin Park, Radwa Barakat, Alexander Ulanov, Zhong Li, Po-Ching Lin, Karen Chiu, Sherry Zhou, Pablo Perez, Jungyeon Lee, Jodi Flaws, CheMyong Jay Ko,Sanitary pads and diapers contain higher phthalate contents than those in common commercial plastic products, Reproductive Toxicology. 2019; 84:114–121. https://doi.org/10.1016/j.reprotox.2019.01.005

Nutrition

Goldin BR, Adlercreutz H, Gorbach SL, Warram JH, Dwyer JT, Swenson L, Woods MN. Estrogen excretion patterns and plasma levels in vegetarian and omnivorous women. N Engl J Med. 1982 Dec 16;307(25):1542-7. doi: 10.1056/NEJM198212163072502. PMID: 7144835

Gorbach SL, Goldin BR. Diet and the excretion and enterohepatic cycling of estrogens. Prev Med. 1987 Jul;16(4):525-31. doi: 10.1016/0091-7435(87)90067-3.PMID: 3628202

Reddy BS, Hanson D, Mangat S, Mathews L, Sbaschnig M, Sharma C, Simi B. Effect of high-fat, high-beef diet and of mode of cooking of beef in the diet on fecal bacterial enzymes and fecal bile acids and neutral sterols. J Nutr. 1980 Sep;110(9):1880–7. doi: 10.1093/jn/110.9.1880. PMID: 7411244

Domellof L, Darby L, Hanson D, Mathews L, Simi B, Reddy BS. Fecal sterols and bacterial beta-glucuronidase activity: a preliminary metabolic epidemiology study of healthy volunteers from Umea, Sweden, and metropolitan New York. Nutr Cancer. 1982;4(2):120–7. doi: 10.1080/01635588209513747. PMID: 6298751

Y. Handa, H. Fujita, Y. Watanabe, S. Honma, M. Kaneuchi, H. Minakami, and R. Kishi. Does dietary estrogen intake from meat relate to the incidence of hormone-dependent cancers? Journal of Clinical Oncology. 2010;28:15, 1553–1553

Harmon BE, Morimoto Y, Beckford F, Franke AA, Stanczyk FZ, Maskarinec G. Oestrogen levels in serum and urine of premenopausal women eating low and high amounts of meat. Public Health Nutr. 2014;17(9):2087–2093. PMID: 24050121

Sánchez-Zamorano LM, Flores-Luna L, Angeles-Llerenas A, Ortega-Olvera C, Lazcano-Ponce E, Romieu I, Mainero-Ratchelous F, Torres-Mejía G. The Western dietary pattern is associated with increased serum concentrations of free estradiol in postmenopausal women: implications for breast cancer prevention. Nutr Res. 2016 Aug;36(8):845–54. Epub 2016, Apr 26. PMID: 27440539

Samsel A, Seneff S. Glyphosate, pathways to modern diseases II: Celiac sprue and gluten intolerance. Interdiscip Toxicol. 2013;6(4):159–184. doi:10.2478/intox-2013–0026

Tempkin A, Naidenko O. Glyphosate Contamination in Food Goes Far Beyond Oat Products. Environmental Working Group. Published February 28, 2019. Accessed July 21, 2021. https://www.ewg.org/news-insights/news/glyphosate-contamination-food-goes-far-beyond-oat-products

Stress

Jenny Gu, Clara Strauss, Rod Bond, Kate Cavanagh. How do mindfulness-based cognitive therapy and mindfulness-based stress reduction improve mental health and wellbeing? A systematic review and meta-analysis of mediation studies. Clinical Psychology Review. 2015;37:1–12. https://doi.org/10.1016/j.cpr.2015.01.006

Bassam Khoury, Tania Lecomte, Guillaume Fortin, Marjolaine Masse, Phillip Therien, Vanessa Bouchard, Marie-Andrée Chapleau, Karine Paquin, Stefan G. Hofmann. Mindfulness-based therapy: A comprehensive meta-analysis. Clinical Psychology Review. 2013;33(6):763–771. https://doi.org/10.1016/j.cpr.2013.05.005

Huberty J, Green J, Glissmann C, Larkey L, Puzia M, Lee C. Efficacy of the Mindfulness Meditation Mobile App "Calm" to Reduce Stress Among College Students: Randomized Controlled Trial. JMIR Mhealth Uhealth 2019;7(6):e14273. doi: 10.2196/14273. PMID: 31237569

Shohani M, Badfar G, Nasirkandy MP, et al. The Effect of Yoga on Stress, Anxiety, and Depression in Women. Int J Prev Med. 2018;9:21. Published 2018 Feb 21. doi:10.4103/ijpvm.IJPVM_242_16. PMID: 29541436

Sharma M. Yoga as an alternative and complementary approach for stress management: a systematic review. J Evid Based Complementary Altern Med. 2014 Jan;19(1):59–67. doi: 10.1177/2156587213503344. Epub 2013 Sep 12. PMID: 24647380

Ma X, Yue ZQ, Gong ZQ, et al. The Effect of Diaphragmatic Breathing on Attention, Negative Affect and Stress in Healthy Adults. Front Psychol. 2017;8:874. Published 2017 Jun 6. doi:10.3389/fpsyg.2017.00874. PMID: 28626434

Hamasaki H. Effects of Diaphragmatic Breathing on Health: A Narrative Review. Medicines (Basel). 2020;7(10):65. Published 2020 Oct 15. doi:10.3390/medicines7100065. PMID: 33076360

Sinatra ST, Oschman JL, Chevalier G, Sinatra D. Electric Nutrition: The Surprising Health and Healing Benefits of Biological Grounding (Earthing). Altern Ther Health Med. 2017 Sep;23(5):8–16. PMID: 28987038

Menigoz W, Latz TT, Ely RA, Kamei C, Melvin G, Sinatra D. Integrative and lifestyle medicine strategies should include Earthing (grounding): Review of research evidence and clinical observations. Explore. 2020 May–Jun;16(3):152–160. doi: 10.1016/j.explore.2019.10.005. Epub 2019 Nov 14. PMID: 31831261

Sleep

Conor J Wild, Emily S Nichols, Michael E Battista, Bobby Stojanoski, Adrian M Owen. Dissociable effects of self-reported daily sleep duration on high-level cognitive abilities. Sleep, 2018; DOI: 10.1093/sleep/zsy182

Watson NF, Badr MS, Belenky G, et al. Recommended Amount of Sleep for a Healthy Adult: A Joint Consensus Statement of the American Academy of Sleep Medicine and Sleep Research Society. Sleep. 2015;38(6):843–844. Published 2015 Jun 1. doi:10.5665/sleep.4716. PMID: 26039963

Yeager, Ronnie & Oleske, Deanna & Sanders, Ruth & Watkins, John & Eells, Janis & Henshel, Diane. (2007). Melatonin as a principal component of red light therapy. Medical hypotheses. 69. 372–6. 10.1016/j.mehy.2006.12.041. Barsam T, Monazzam MR, Haghdoost AA, Ghotbi MR, Dehghan SF. Effect of extremely low frequency electromagnetic field exposure on sleep quality in high voltage substations. Iranian J Environ Health Sci Eng. 2012;9(1):15. Published 2012 Nov 30. doi:10.1186/1735-2746-9-15. PMID: 23369281

Liu H, Chen G, Pan Y, Chen Z, Jin W, Sun C, et al. (2014) Occupational Electromagnetic Field Exposures Associated with Sleep Quality: A Cross-Sectional Study. PLoS ONE 9(10): e110825. https://doi.org/10.1371/journal.pone.0110825

Chaput JP, Tremblay A. Adequate sleep to improve the treatment of obesity. CMAJ. 2012;184(18):1975–1976. doi:10.1503/cmaj.120876. PMID: 22988148

Schmid SM, Hallschmid M, Jauch-Chara K, Born J, Schultes B. A single night of sleep deprivation increases ghrelin levels and feelings of hunger in normal-weight healthy men. J Sleep Res. 2008 Sep;17(3):331–4. doi: 10.1111/j.1365-2869.2008.00662.x. Epub 2008 Jun 28. PMID: 18564298

Christine Blume, Corrado Garbazza, Manuel Spitschan. Effects of light on human circadian rhythms, sleep and mood. Somnologie (Berl). 2019; 23(3): 147–156. doi: 10.1007/s11818-019-00215-x. PMID: 31534436

Zhao J, Tian Y, Nie J, Xu J, Liu D. Red light and the sleep quality and endurance performance of Chinese female basketball players. J Athl Train. 2012;47(6):673–678. doi:10.4085/1062-6050-47.6.08. PMID: 23182016

Natural Remedies

Yablon LA, Mauskop A. Magnesium in headache. In: Vink R, Nechifor M, editors. Magnesium in the Central Nervous System [Internet]. Adelaide (AU): University of Adelaide Press; 2011. Available from: https://www.ncbi.nlm.nih.gov/books/NBK507271/

Abdolahi M, Jafarieh A, Sarraf P, Sedighiyan M, Yousefi A, Tafakhori A, Abdollahi H, Salehinia F, Djalali M. The Neuromodulatory Effects of ω-3 Fatty Acids and Nano-Curcumin on the COX-2/ iNOS Network in Migraines: A Clinical Trial Study from Gene Expression to Clinical Symptoms. Endocr Metab Immune Disord Drug Targets. 2019;19(6):874–884. doi: 10.2174/1871530319666190212170140. PMID: 30760195

Maghbooli M, Golipour F, Moghimi Esfandabadi A, Yousefi M. Comparison between the efficacy of ginger and sumatriptan in the ablative treatment of the common migraine. Phytother Res. 2014 Mar;28(3):412–5. doi: 10.1002/ptr.4996. Epub 2013 May 9. PMID: 23657930

Martins LB, Rodrigues AMDS, Rodrigues DF, Dos Santos LC, Teixeira AL, Ferreira AVM. Double-blind placebo-controlled randomized clinical trial of ginger (Zingiber officinale Rosc.) addition in migraine acute treatment. Cephalalgia. 2019 Jan;39(1):68–76. doi: 10.1177/0333102418776016. Epub 2018 May 16. PMID: 29768938

Sasannejad P, Saeedi M, Shoeibi A, Gorji A, Abbasi M, Foroughipour M. Lavender essential oil in the treatment of migraine headache: a placebo-controlled clinical trial. Eur Neurol. 2012;67(5):288–91. doi: 10.1159/000335249. Epub 2012 Apr 17. PMID: 22517298

Supplements

Rajoria S, Suriano R, Parmar PS, et al. 3,3'-diindolylmethane modulates estrogen metabolism in patients with thyroid proliferative disease: a pilot study. Thyroid. 2011;21(3):299–304. doi:10.1089/thy.2010.0245

Dalessandri KM, Firestone GL, Fitch MD, Bradlow HL, Bjeldanes LF. Pilot study: effect of 3,3'-diindolylmethane supplements on urinary hormone metabolites in postmenopausal women with a history of early-stage breast cancer. Nutr Cancer. 2004;50(2):161–7. doi: 10.1207/s15327914nc5002_5. PMID: 15623462

Rinat Yerushalmi, Sharon Bargil, Yaara Ber, Rachel Ozlavo, Tuval Sivan, Yael Rapson, Adi Pomerantz, Daliah Tsoref, Eran Sharon, Opher Caspi, Ahuvah Grubsrein, David Margel, 3,3-Diindolylmethane (DIM): a nutritional intervention and its impact on breast density in healthy BRCA carriers. A prospective clinical trial, Carcinogenesis, Volume 41, Issue 10, October 2020, Pages 1395–1401, https://doi.org/10.1093/carcin/bgaa050

Auborn KJ, Fan S, Rosen EM, Goodwin L, Chandraskaren A, Williams DE, Chen D, Carter TH. Indole-3-carbinol is a negative regulator of estrogen. J Nutr. 2003 Jul;133(7 Suppl):2470S-2475S. doi: 10.1093/jn/133.7.2470s. PMID: 12840226

Nguyen HH, Lavrenov SN, Sundar SN, Nguyen DH, Tseng M, Marconett CN, Kung J, Staub RE, Preobrazhenskaya MN, Bjeldanes LF, Firestone GL. 1-Benzyl-indole-3-carbinol is a novel indole-3-carbinol derivative with significantly enhanced potency of anti-proliferative and anti-estrogenic properties in human breast cancer cells. Chem Biol Interact. 2010 Aug 5;186(3):255–66. doi: 10.1016/j.cbi.2010.05.015. Epub 2010 Jun 2. PMID: 20570586; PMCID: PMC3422669

Calcium-D-glucarate. Altern Med Rev. 2002 Aug;7(4):336–9. PMID: 12197785

Abraham GE. Nutritional factors in the etiology of the premenstrual tension syndromes. J Reprod Med. 1983 Jul;28(7):446–64. PMID: 6684167

Danielius Serapinas, Evelina Boreikaite, Agne Bartkeviciute, Rita Bandzeviciene, Mindaugas Silkunas, Daiva Bartkeviciene. The importance of folate, vitamins B6 and B12 for the lowering of homocysteine concentrations for patients with recurrent pregnancy loss and MTHFR mutations. Reproductive Toxicology. 2017;72:159-163. https://doi.org/10.1016/j.reprotox.2017.07.001

van Die MD, Burger HG, Teede HJ, Bone KM. Vitex agnus-castus extracts for female reproductive disorders: a systematic review of clinical trials. Planta Med. 2013 May;79(7):562–75. doi: 10.1055/s-0032-1327831. Epub 2012 Nov 7. PMID: 23136064

Wuttke W, Jarry H, Christoffel V, Spengler B, Seidlová-Wuttke D. Chaste tree (Vitex agnus-castus)—pharmacology and clinical indications. Phytomedicine. 2003 May;10(4):348–57. doi: 10.1078/094471103322004866. PMID: 12809367

Mahboubi M. Evening Primrose (Oenothera biennis) Oil in Management of Female Ailments. J Menopausal Med. 2019;25(2):74–82. doi:10.6118/jmm.18190

Skibola CF. The effect of Fucus vesiculosus, an edible brown seaweed, upon menstrual cycle length and hormonal status in three pre-menopausal women: a case report. BMC Complement Altern Med. 2004;4:10. Published 2004 Aug 4. doi:10.1186/1472-6882-4-10. PMID: 15294021

Chandrasekhar K, Kapoor J, Anishetty S. A prospective, randomized double-blind, placebo-controlled study of safety and efficacy of a high-concentration full-spectrum extract of ashwagandha root in reducing stress and anxiety in adults. Indian J Psychol Med. 2012;34(3):255–262. doi:10.4103/0253-7176.106022. PMID: 23439798

Ion-George Anghelescu, David Edwards, Erich Seifritz & Siegfried Kasper (2018) Stress management and the role of Rhodiola rosea: a review. International Journal of Psychiatry in Clinical Practice. 22:4,242–252, DOI: 10.1080/13651501.2017.1417442

Ahn J, Ahn HS, Cheong JH, Dela Peña I. Natural Product-Derived Treatments for Attention-Deficit/Hyperactivity Disorder: Safety, Efficacy, and Therapeutic Potential of Combination Therapy. Neural Plast. 2016;2016:1320423. doi:10.1155/2016/1320423. PMID: 26966583

Cohen MM. Tulsi—Ocimum sanctum: A herb for all reasons. J Ayurveda Integr Med. 2014;5(4):251–259. doi:10.4103/0975-9476.146554. PMID: 25624701

Calabrese C, Gregory WL, Leo M, Kraemer D, Bone K, Oken B. Effects of a standardized Bacopa monnieri extract on cognitive performance, anxiety, and depression in the elderly: a randomized, double-blind, placebo-controlled trial. J Altern Complement Med. 2008;14(6):707–713. doi:10.1089/acm.2008.0018. PMID: 18611150

Camfield DA, Wetherell MA, Scholey AB, et al. The effects of multivitamin supplementation on diurnal cortisol secretion and perceived stress. Nutrients. 2013;5(11):4429–4450. Published 2013 Nov 11. doi:10.3390/nu5114429. PMID: 24284609

Patak P, Willenberg HS, Bornstein SR. Vitamin C is an important cofactor for both adrenal cortex and adrenal medulla. Endocr Res. 2004 Nov;30(4):871–5. doi: 10.1081/erc-200044126. PMID: 15666839

Khoshbaten M, Aliasgarzadeh A, Masnadi K, et al. N-acetylcysteine improves liver function in patients with non-alcoholic Fatty liver disease. Hepat Mon. 2010;10(1):12–16. PMID: 22308119

Chen X. Protective effects of quercetin on liver injury induced by ethanol. Pharmacogn Mag. 2010;6(22):135–141. doi:10.4103/0973-1296.62900. PMID: 20668581

Mulrow C, Lawrence V, Jacobs B, et al. Milk Thistle: Effects on Liver Disease and Cirrhosis and Clinical Adverse Effects: Summary. 2000. AHRQ Evidence Report Summaries. Rockville (MD): Agency for Healthcare Research and Quality (US); 1998–2005. 21. Available from: https://www.ncbi.nlm.nih.gov/books/NBK11896/

Devaraj, Ezhilarasan. Hepatoprotective properties of Dandelion: Recent update. Journal of Applied Pharmaceutical Science. (2016)6. 202–205. 10.7324/JAPS.2016.60429

Printed in Great Britain
by Amazon